You will find this book helpful if you are experiencing any of the following symptoms.

- Gastro-intestinal problems, including tummy aches, bloating, diarrhoea, loose stools, constipation, wind and Irritable Bowel Syndrome.
- Headaches or migraines.
- Skin conditions, including eczema, rashes, itching and adult acne.
- Asthma, catarrh or cough, including rhinitis and throat clearing.
- Fatigue, anxiety and depression, including panic attacks.
- Child behaviour problems.

Reading this book will help you if you:

- suffer from any of the symptoms above and feel traditional medical treatment is not helping;
- suspect you have a food intolerance, but cannot work out what it might be;
- are seeking alternatives to medication to deal with the symptoms;
- are interested in how and why the foods to which people react have changed in recent years.

The book details the most likely foods and drinks that people are intolerant of, according to data collected by the author from clients seen between 2003 and 2015. She gives detailed recommendations for how to avoid these foods.

Each of the most common symptoms of food intolerance has a dedicated chapter. This will help you understand the food intolerance causes, triggers and recommended solutions.

Each chapter includes real-life case studies, as well as data and relevant information about food intolerance patterns in 2015.

Further chapters explain common misconceptions about:

- cow's milk and lactose;
- wheat or yeast;
- alcohol;
- artificial flavouring; and
- supposedly healthy 'clean' eating.

What people are saying about Mary...

Testimonial from a local general practitioner

Mary helped me when I had bilateral frozen shoulders. I have a full range of movement following Mary's recommended change of diet. I refer many of my patients with Irritable Bowel Syndrome, eczema, fatigue or non-arthritic joint symptoms to Mary. I know many have been helped.

FQ [Sutton General Practitioner]

Ulcerative colitis

My visit to Mary in 2014 literally changed my life. I was diagnosed with ulcerative colitis in 2008, and had been on steroids, which had bad side effects, and did not help my symptoms. Doctors said that I would need to be on medication for the rest of my life, and there was no known cause. Within four days of cutting dairy, oranges and coffee out of my diet I came off all medication. My colitis is now in remission and has been ever since. Even better, I was able to have a small amount of cheese at Christmas with no negative effects! Thank you Mary.

Anonymous

Migraine

I was struggling every day with severe headache, migraine, Irritable Bowel and catarrh symptoms, and I needed help to identify and clarify which foods I was intolerant to. I found Mary very knowledgeable and helpful giving me food alternatives I could try. The visit to Mary gave me my life back and several people told me I was like a different person. I have also had to visit Mary with my five year old son, and she has offered great after care advice too. I would recommend Mary to anyone who is struggling with migraines.

Michele Jeffries [Southampton]

Tummy pain, bloating, fatigue, headache and mood swings

Before visiting Mary, I had felt ill for more than a year and was getting worse each week. I had constant stomach cramp, fatigue, headaches, mood swings and felt bloated all the time. Within four weeks my symptoms had almost disappeared and I felt uplifted. Eight weeks after my first testing I was running three or four times a week. I even managed a 5k run! Thank you so much Mary.

Chrissy [Sutton]

Abdominal pain, nausea, knee pain and cough

After three years of 'Hell' including endoscopy twice, barium meal test, X-Rays, blood tests and hypnotherapy, I found Mary following an enquiry in a health food shop. I was nauseated, constantly retching, and suffering severe abdominal pain. Even close relatives thought my nausea was 'in my head'. My testing showed that I was intolerant to dairy products, malt, orange and sunflower.

I had spent hundreds of pounds over three years, yet two hours with Mary for a very small amount of money and I was cured within four days. An added bonus was no more pain in my knees. I went back to Mary again recently. I had developed new intolerances which were the cause of my coughing for the previous years. Again, doctors and X-Rays had not been able to solve my problem. Thank you Mary, you are a star!

Julie [Carshalton]

Adult acne

I suffered from facial acne for most of my teens and well into my adult life. I had been prescribed the pill, antibiotics and topical lotions all to no avail. I dreaded social occasions and even going to work on some days when my skin was at its worst.

Mary told me I was intolerant to cheese and chocolate, both which I ate on a daily basis! Since cutting them out of my diet my skin has cleared!

These days I will eat the odd main course containing cheese and maybe the odd chocolate, but neither to the extent I used to eat. I certainly wish I had known about Mary years ago!

P Tait [Sutton]

Throat clearing and bloating

After years of putting up with on/off bloating and throat clearing, I decided to seek help from Mary, who was friendly and professional. I had a few intolerances, dairy products, grass pollen, chemical fragrances and feathers. I removed all these (apart from the grass pollen!) and it has changed my life. No more bloating or throat clearing. Impressive.

A Newman [Epsom]

Migraine and headache

1. No more headaches or migraine after having suffered them for 20 years.
2. All possible causes dealt with, and I had no idea that many of these would have any impact [Chemicals in regular products, blood sugar levels, vitamin status].
3. I needed a second test one week later as I was not completely better. No charge for this, and this is Mary's standard service for any client.
4. Completely free email and phone back up.
5. A thoroughly sympathetic service. She takes time to really understand where you are coming from and really listens.

JD [Purley]

Attention deficit hyperactivity disorder

Thank you Mary. You have given our family our life back. We have not had to start Jake on Ritalin after all. He seems like a different boy since avoiding dairy and sweet artificial flavours. His teachers have commented that he can concentrate well, and he seems at last to be capable of making friends. 'Mr Angry' has gone away! Thank you so much.

Kate [Reigate]

Acne

I saw Mary at the age of 20 after having suffered facial acne and acne scarring for the best part of five years. Having had various allergy tests and tried medications to reduce the acne, nothing worked. Cutting down dairy products had helped before I met Mary. Confirmation of this intolerance, and carefully avoiding orange and sunflower provided so much relief. I was no longer embarrassed by my acne, and my confidence was back. Without Mary I would not be as happy, and I am so grateful. Thank you!!

Charlotte [Purley]

Abdominal pain, headache, asthma, joint pain, sinus pain, deafness

For many years I had suffered from intestinal problems, headaches, asthma, sinus pain, deafness in one ear and severe aching joints. I had been thoroughly investigated via the NHS. Mary found that I reacted to all animal milk products, household chemicals, oranges, mould and aspartame. By the end of the first week all my family and friends could not believe the change in me. The increase in energy, life without pain, no intestinal problems, and I could hear again. Mary has changed my life. I cannot believe that allergy testing could make so much difference. If I had been tested earlier the NHS would have saved a lot of money. I have recommended Mary to many friends and family and all of them have had very good results. The in depth information Mary gives you as to why and how your body develops an intolerance is fascinating.

PM   [Hayes, Kent]

Irritable Bowel Syndrome, aches and pains

I saw Mary in June last year when I was in the UK visiting family from Australia. Prior to seeing her, I had suffered with stomach pain, being bloated, feeling generally unwell with aches and pains. I had tried to diagnose myself, and had cut out so many things from my diet that I had stopped enjoying food altogether. And I still was unwell. I had resigned myself to having invasive testing done in Australia. After cutting dairy (the culprit) out of my diet, my stomach pain and all the other symptoms disappeared. I felt amazing in a very short space of time. Now, nearly seven months later I am very used to my change of diet and feel healthier than I have felt in about three years. I can't thank Mary enough for helping me when she did.

Eczema

I took my two year old to see Mary because of his severe eczema. We had seen GPs and two dermatologists all to no avail. Tom was miserable... and so were we! His eczema was on his face, arms, legs, torso and in his ears. Testing showed that Tom was intolerant to dairy products, and apple, both of which he loved. Within a week of avoiding the foods Tom's skin was no longer itchy, and within a fortnight his skin was clear. Mary advised that we give Tom zinc drops, change the products we wash his clothes in, and use a different shampoo. Why isn't this service available on the NHS?

Sharon [Wallington]

Acknowledgements

I am not a natural 'gusher', but please take it as read that my thanks to the following family and friends are heart-felt and your help has been massively appreciated.

- My husband John, who has been immensely supportive in keeping the home fires burning and encouraging me when I have had to perform tasks which were way out of my comfort zone.
- My adult boys, Pete, Will and Steve and Pete's partner Bea, who have all given me ideas and helped with computers, online appointment bookings, social networking tips, book titles and ways of changing a business which has become too busy.
- My good friend Liz Stopani who has been the best listener and sounding board.
- Chris Day, Director of Filament Publishing, who has been helpful and generous far beyond the call of duty and endlessly patient with me when he has suggested tasks which have worried me a great deal.
- My editor, book and business coach, Wendy Yorke who has pulled and pushed my ramblings into a cohesive whole, whilst at the same time being marvellously encouraging.

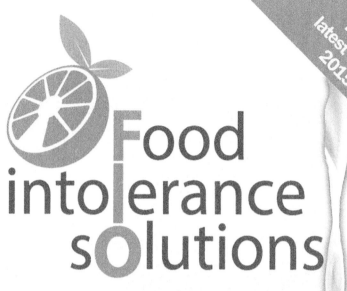

Food intolerance solutions

Proven solutions for relief from headache, migraine, IBS, catarrh, rhinitis, asthma, eczema, rashes, acne, fatigue and child behaviour problems

Including the latest data from the 2015 Survey

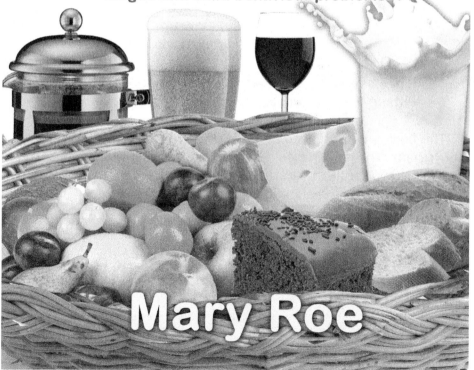

Mary Roe

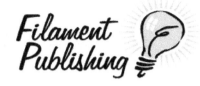

Published by
Filament Publishing Ltd
16 Croydon Road, Beddington, Croydon,
Surrey, CR0 4PA, United Kingdom.
+44(0)20 8688 2598
www.filamentpublishing.com

ISBN 978-1-910819-93-7

Printed by IngramSpark

This book is not intended as a substitute for the medical advice of
physicians. The reader should regularly consult a physician in matters
relating to his/her health and particularly with respect to any symptoms
that may require diagnosis or medical attention.

Contents

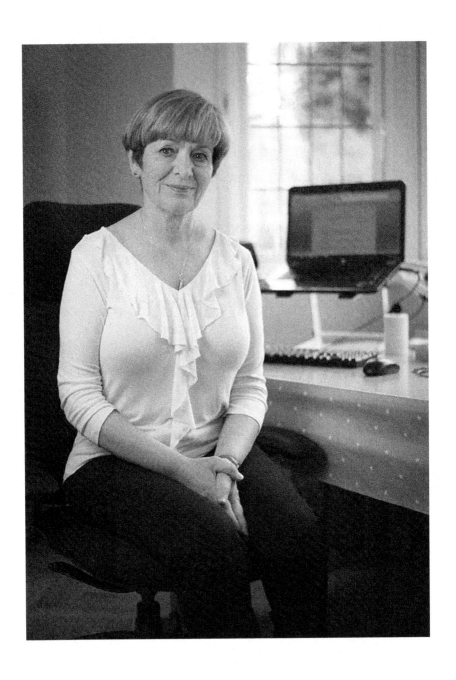

About Mary Roe

Ly introduction to food intolerance came 30 years ago, when my husband and I were struggling to cope with our two oldest children. Before this, I had the typical NHS mentality that food intolerance was just a trendy fad but I experienced a complete sea-change.

Our oldest child was four years old, and by midday every day had a rock hard, distended tummy, about the size of a seven month pregnancy. He had two different sizes of trousers to accommodate his daily increase in girth.

One day he had a tummy bug, and did not eat for a few days. His tummy did not swell on those days, so I started wondering, and as a result removed dairy products from my son's diet. I was lucky. I chose the right food. Peter no longer had a bloated tummy, and there was another added benefit. My stroppy, antagonistic four year old was much nicer to be with.

At the same time we were reeling from being told that our baby daughter had a severe learning disability. She was just coming up to her first birthday. She rarely slept, constantly cried, had diarrhoea, and a nose that dripped green catarrh. She was waiting for surgery to have grommets inserted, because her catarrh was affecting her hearing. By the time she was nine months old, Katy had been prescribed 17 courses of antibiotics, for ear infections, chest infections and pneumonia.

I did some research and put her on the 'Stone Age Diet'. This meant feeding Katy on foods that she rarely ate, and by so doing removed all the most common food intolerances from her diet. By day three she was a different baby - happy, smiling, sleeping more soundly – with normal stools. By day seven her nose had cleared, and wonder of wonders, she could hear. I started reintroducing staple foods individually until we found the main culprits. She still had a learning disability, but the picture was very different from the one painted by her paediatrician.

Having achieved such life-changing results from dietary change, it subsequently became a passion of mine - to find out more about food intolerance. Then - ten years later I had the opportunity to start working as a food intolerance tester - and I grasped the chance with both hands.

I bought a franchise in a UK-wide food intolerance testing business. This involved being trained in the use of a Vega machine during a period of six months. There was little other training given but gradually over the years I became proficient in the use of the machine. As my experience grew I was able to give increasingly detailed advice from genuine experience.

I had the start of a good little business, which grew gradually by word of mouth. In 2000 I sold my franchise, and started up on my own. I started following clients up to see how well the exclusion diet was working, and collecting data to see if there were any patterns connecting certain foods to symptoms. It is from the depth of my experience and my many years of client studies and annual surveys that this book is written.

Foreword

At the Surrey Institute of Clinical Hypnotherapy we see thousands of clients every year who have a myriad of psychological and physical problems. Sometimes the client may have physical issues that underlie their problems. As hypnotherapists, although we can sometimes affect the physical aspects of the body (IBS and psoriasis) in the main, we are working with the subconscious mind to change behaviours. If there are underlying medical factors to the clients' problems this can create a brick wall that we cannot get round, under or over. One example is anxiety. A client may come to us to resolve his anxiety issues. One of the key effects of that anxiety is he feels sick. He is anxious because he feels sick. Which comes first, the anxiety or the nausea?

It was in an attempt to solve one such problem that I first referred to Mary Roe. My anxiety client had been feeling sick for three years. The client was intolerant to orange in any form [fruit, juice, squash or peel]. Three days after excluding orange she was no longer feeling sick and was completely anxiety free. Since then I have sent many clients to Mary and she has delivered every time. I have no hesitation in recommending her.

Paul Howard
Principal, Surrey Institute of Hypnotherapy

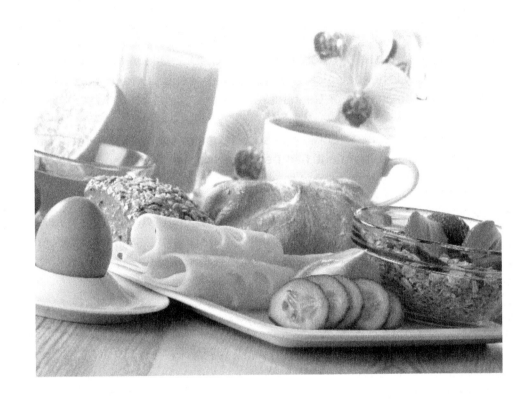

Part 1: Food Intolerance Overview

Chapter 1: Improving your quality of life

I am privileged to work in a field where I help people recover from chronic symptoms, which massively and adversely affect their quality of life.

For example, take Teri, who suffered from debilitating migraines for 30 years, since the birth of her first child. Her only migraine free periods were during two later pregnancies. Since nearing the menopause, Teri's migraines had increased from approximately once a month [premenstrual] to at least once a week. She was unable to work on these days and her usual painkillers were no longer 'nipping it in the bud'. Within ten days of our first meeting, Teri was bright eyed and feeling wonderful. She had no headaches or migraines and since working with me, her fatigue had improved on average by 90%. She went back to work full-time and was enjoying her life again.

Or think about Noelle, an elderly lady who rarely left her house because of urgent diarrhoea. She never knew when it might strike and she had taken to wearing incontinence products 'just in case'. Within three days of avoiding the foods I recommended, Noelle had normal bowel function and felt her life had begun again.

How about Valentina, a 30 year old woman whose adult acne was greatly affecting her confidence. Ten days after a change of diet and vitamin supplementation, Valentina's skin was smooth and blemish free. She was amazed that the dietary change also enabled her to sleep right through the night regularly, for the first time in ten years.

Or Steve, a once fit builder, whose joint and muscle pain meant he could no longer work. My recommended change of diet, which excluded his beloved bread, resulted in a pain free existence. An added bonus for him was his nearly lifelong catarrh problem disappeared.

Also, there was Ethan, who at the tender age of six was struggling with his school work because of his inability to concentrate. He was unable to make friends because of his mood swings. He was driving his parents mad with his inability to listen and his desire to constantly interrupt conversations. A much calmer boy emerged with a change of diet and even more improvements were noticed when he started taking vitamin and mineral supplements.

Eloise was a very sad little two year old with severe eczema, who seemed to undergo a personality change with a change of diet, as well as totally clearing up her skin problems.

I am a registered nurse and I have worked in the field of food intolerance for the last 21 years. Most of my knowledge has been gained through direct experience, a questioning mind and evidence through the analysis of client data. Until 2010, most of my clients came to me by word of mouth recommendation. I had built a good local reputation and gained more than 16 years experience.

When I started building my own website in 2010, I had no idea how my business would expand. I worked hard to build my professional credibility by conducting patient surveys and publishing the data on my website. This brought me many more clients and also had another unexpected effect. I started receiving emails from around the world, asking for my advice about which foods might be causing a person's chronic symptoms.

And the seed of an idea for this book was sown.

Many books have been written about food allergy and food intolerance, mostly documenting symptoms, the likely causes and the common foods which can be involved in reactions. Some of these books are scientific, others are intended for the layperson. Some are anecdotal, including individual accounts of how avoiding certain foods has helped to alleviate symptoms.

The gold standard for detecting food intolerances has for many decades been the elimination diet. Many books have been written suggesting which foods to avoid. The premise behind elimination diets is to avoid all foods that might be a cause of the symptoms for a few weeks, until you have no adverse symptoms. Then you reintroduce those foods individually in a structured way, watching for the symptoms to return. This method enables you to find out which are your problem foods and therefore which foods or drinks to avoid to feel well.

These books lists many foods for you to avoid, including cow's milk products, wheat, yeast, tea, coffee, all alcohol, most additives, citrus fruits, tomatoes, egg, spices, fizzy drinks and sometimes more, depending on their focus.

These elimination diets are difficult to follow and the restrictions often put people off even attempting a start. The process is prolonged, as later reintroduction of individual foods and drinks has to be managed slowly and carefully every three days or so. These books describe the elimination and reintroduction method in detail. At least half of the space in such books is taken up by recipes because the difficulties of following elimination diets make 'normal' eating patterns nearly impossible.

When you read a book, article, website or blog about the elimination diet, you will find that avoidance of certain foods is mentioned many times. And General Practitioners will often advise patients to avoid certain food groups. Many of my clients have dabbled with avoiding these foods. They are really surprised when on testing I tell them that the food is not a part of their problem because they have been led to believe these are foods which are likely causes of their symptoms. The chart below details these foods and the incidence of how often a person is intolerant to them on testing.

Data from my 2015 Survey of 441 people

Food	Percentage of adults	Percentage of children
Dairy products	35	70
Alcohol	10	n/a
Orange	28	42
Other citrus fruits	>2	none
Wheat	>1	>1
Egg	>1	none
Tomato	>1	none
Other foods from nightshade family e.g. potato, peppers, aubergine	>1	none
Nitrates and nitrites	>0.5	none
Sulphites in wine	>0.5	n/a
Sulphates in dried fruit	none	none
Onions	none	none

How I test my clients

I use a Dietx machine to test which foods and products are adversely affecting my clients. The Dietx machine is the latest model of the Vega machine. Dietx and the Vega machines work on the same principles. They are galvanometers, and act as a resistance-measuring instrument via an electrical circuit. The person being tested holds onto a metal cylinder which is connected to the machine. The tester uses a probe to touch an acupuncture point close to the client's finger nail, toenail or the palm of their hand, completing the circuit. The tester has many vials of foods and drinks, which are placed one by one in the machine. A dial on the machine gives a marked low reading when a food/drink/product is adversely affecting the person being tested.

The Vega and Dietx machines can be very useful tools, provided the operator has sufficient experience to produce reliable and consistent results. The two day training course provided in the UK when someone buys the Dietx machine is not sufficient for an operator to ensure reliable results. Reliability and consistency take months of diligent practice. Just as important as knowing how to operate the machine, is the structured process of questioning by which the tester finds the root of the client's problems and an understanding of which foods/drinks might be potential intolerances.

The contents of the testing vials sold with the Dietx machine in 2015/16 has not been changed or added to since the 1980s. Changes in eating habits mean there are new foods/drinks/additives people react to in 2015. These foods are not yet in the Dietx testing kit, which means that most testers do not test them. But I do! For more information read *Chapter 14: Supposedly healthy 'clean' eating.*

Using the data I have collected from testing my clients since 2003, plus my 21 years of experience, I recommend an exclusion diet for you based on your symptoms, age and gender. For more information read *Chapter 15: Recommended diet for your age and gender.*

For several symptoms, I suggest you change the products you are using to wash your clothes or fragrance your home. For other symptoms I recommend adding vitamin or mineral supplements to your diet.

Few doctors, health workers or alternative health practitioners know exactly how well their methods work, in regard to symptomatic improvement in their clients. In 2012, I decided I needed evidence of how successful my methods were and I started surveying my clients. It is this detailed information which I share with you in this book and which demonstrates the positive results I have experienced.

Symptom Improvement Survey 2012

This survey was based on the responses of 236 clients to a questionnaire sent approximately four to six weeks after starting my recommended diet. Clients were asked, what percentage of improvement for each of their symptoms they had experienced by changing their diet, from 100%, 95%, 90%, 80%, 65%, under 65%, or no improvement.

Symptom	Average percentage improvement
Bloating	86
Abdominal pain	92 [98 in children]
Diarrhoea	98
Loose stools	95
Wind	83
Constipation	89
Urgency to defaecate	99
Indigestion	100
Nausea	98
Vomiting	100
Headache	95
Migraine	100
Eczema	94 [97 in children]
Rash	85 [96 in children]
Itch	99
Acne	91
Catarrh	83 [90 in children]
Asthma	84
Frequent colds	87
Persistent cough	100
Fatigue	95
Lethargy	98
Children's behaviour, mood swings	88

This book has a second strand. There are several myths about food intolerance, which have become so well known in the media that they are masquerading as the truth. These myths have spread into the public consciousness gradually because they are repeated on the radio and on television, as well as in newspapers, magazines, online articles, blogs and additional online forums. In this book, I am suggesting, with reference to the data that I have gathered, that many of these 'truths' are actually fallacies and rumours.

This book addresses the following misconceptions.

- Is wheat a common food intolerance?
- Are lactose and cow's milk the same thing?
- Is it healthier for you to use decaffeinated products?
- Is intolerance to additives more common than intolerance to staple healthy foods?

The foods people react most commonly to are subtly changing as the years go by. I have evidence to demonstrate that the foods earmarked as being common intolerances between ten and 30 years ago are problematic to a lower percentage of people now. Several foods are more commonly a problem now than 30 years ago. Read more about this in *Chapter 2: Food intolerance synopsis* and in *Chapter 14: Supposedly healthy 'clean' eating.*

Chapter 2: Food intolerance synopsis

There is one pattern which is really important to understand in relation to food intolerance. The most likely food reactions will be to frequently used foods and drinks. To become intolerant of a food or drink it is likely to be consumed at least twice daily. It does not matter how much volume is taken on each occasion, but the number of times a day the food/drink is consumed. Cow's milk products are a common food intolerance in the western hemisphere, but not in the Far East, where soya or rice are more commonly implicated.

Think about your daily diet. Which foods or drinks do you have more than twice a day?

The reason people find it difficult to work out for themselves what their problem foods are, is because their symptoms are similar from day to day, or they are experienced in clusters. Keeping a food diary rarely seems to clarify things for the sufferer. In fact, diary keeping often does little more than make the person restrict more foods, which actually are not the causes of their problems. This is especially the case when digestive symptoms are involved. Symptoms can occur a few minutes or a few days after eating a problem food. It is very difficult to work it out on your own. Frequent consumption of a staple food or drink is usually the underlying problem, but the sufferer presumes the food most recently eaten is the cause. For more information read *Chapter 4: Gastro-intestinal and digestion*.

Case Study
Esther was convinced spices, fruit, vegetables and fizzy drinks affected her tummy adversely. As a result, her diet was bland and not especially healthy. However, after she removed cow's milk products from her diet, she suffered no symptoms from the foods she had suspected previously.

In my 2011 Survey, I demonstrated that people were only 17% accurate in assessing what their problem foods were.

Why you? Why now?

Why is it that a person can be healthy, energetic, able to eat anything without any problem and suddenly suffer from symptoms that massively affect their quality of life?

Reasons why food intolerances start or become worse

Any of the factors below can trigger someone to start reacting to a food which has not affected them before, or cause symptoms already present to worsen.

Viruses, influenza, norovirus, severe infections, tummy bugs, gastroenteritis, salmonella, E coli, sore throats, ear infections, glandular fever
Operations
Hormone changes, e.g. puberty, pregnancy, childbirth, stopping breastfeeding, any form of contraception, [pill, mini pill, merine coil, depo injection, or implant]
Stressful situations e.g. bereavement, divorce, overwork, moving house, severe illness in the family, relationship break-up, bullying at school or in the workplace
Courses of antibiotics, especially long term courses

Case Study
Susannah regularly had migraines pre-menstrually from puberty until she went on the pill aged 21. At that stage her migraines started happening once or twice a week.

Which are the most common food intolerances?

In my 2015 Survey of 345 adults and 96 children, these were the most common food intolerances.

Food	Percentage of adults	Percentage of children
Cow's milk products	35	71
Cocoa	38	39
Yeast, all cheeses and all yogurts	30	>1
Coffee	29	>1
Tea	28	>1
Orange	29	46
Apple	9	30
Sweet artificial flavours	12	12
E150 – E155 dark brown food colouring	12	5
Decaffeinated drinks	12	n/a
Some form of alcohol	10	n/a
Monosodium glutamate	9	9
Aspartame	4	9
Sunflower	6	5
Cheese alone	4	3
Soya	2	2
Wheat	>1	none
Every other food was less than 1%		

Points to note

- The percentage differences for some foods between adults and children is marked. For more information read *Chapter 3: Food intolerance in children.*
- Tea and coffee were only a problem for adults who drank either beverage more than twice a day, or for those who had in the past drunk them more than twice a day and had since reduced the frequency of use. All but 5% of frequent tea and coffee drinkers were intolerant of their favourite beverage.

- An exception to this was when cocoa was the main intolerance. Several chocolate lovers rarely drank coffee, but it would give them similar adverse symptoms because cocoa and coffee beans are very closely related.
- Decaffeinated drinks were responsible for symptoms in only 12% of adults. However, they were all regular consumers of decaffeinated drinks. For more information read *Chapter 14: Supposedly healthy 'clean' eating.*
- Yeast, cheese and yogurt come as a package. When someone is intolerant of yeast, they will almost without exception be intolerant of cheese and yogurt too. Only one adult in the survey was intolerant of yeast alone. All of the others intolerant of yeast, had a problem with all cheeses and all yogurts. The numbers of people reacting to cheese was higher than yeast and yogurt because some people are intolerant of only cheese and not other milk products.
- Although 30% of adults were yeast, cheese and yogurt intolerant, no children under 16 were, and there was only one girl in the 16 - 18 year age bracket.
- The percentage of people with intolerances of the two major food groups; yeast, cheese, yogurt and cow's milk products; was very small at less than 1%. There was only one person.
- 10% of adults were intolerant to some form of alcohol, and this was often, but not always, their favourite drink. Only one person out of 345 had a problem with all alcohol. For more information read *Chapter 13: Alcohol.*
- Chilli was only a problem for people who used it frequently, e.g. people from the Asian community, or those who added it to every meal in the form of e.g. Tabasco, because they loved the heat of it.
- Aspartame was only a problem for people who regularly used it in diet or sugar free drinks, sweets or chewing gums. The incidence was higher in children than adults because of their use of sugar free/no added sugar fruit squashes.
- Apple was part of the picture for those who commonly consumed apples, drank apple juice or squash. It was especially common in babies and toddlers because apple is often used as a sugar substitute in foods dedicated to this age group.

Case Studies

> Danny loved chocolate and was not surprised to discover it was cocoa causing his fatigue and headaches, once I had explained that frequent or favourite foods are often culprits. He was intolerant of coffee as well, even though he only drank it once daily.

> Hayley was intolerant of yeast, cheese and yogurt. She had thought that her problem was wheat, because she knew she had reactions after pasta [always with some grated parmesan], pizza [with cheese on top, and yeast in the pizza base], and bread [contains yeast].

> Maureen drank ten cups of tea a day, and had done so since she was a child in Ireland.

> Darren started drinking decaffeinated coffee when he was finding it hard to get off to sleep at night. Coffee was something he liked to drink through the day and evening, but once he found that the decaffeinated coffee was at the root of his skin problem, he was happy to have his last coffee at 5pm.

Will you be able to eat your problem foods again?
Yes, absolutely, in a large majority of cases!

To get to the stage where you can do this you need to avoid the foods which you react to completely, for at least three months. The stricter you can be in avoiding these foods the better your chances of recovery. The majority of people feel better if they cut down on their problem foods. However, not everyone does. There is no way of knowing which group you or your child might fall into. A complete break from the culprit food is what enables the body to recover. If you are not strict with the exclusion diet, or do not complete the full three months, your body will not recover, and every time you return to normal eating, the same symptoms will return.

I have found that in excess of 90% of adults can eat their problem foods again, without suffering symptoms, after three months exclusion. The figures in children are even better, in excess of 95%. Maybe the difference in these figures is due to the fact that children are 'policed' well by their parents and therefore, do not touch their problem foods for the three months required. Whereas adults cannot manage to avoid foods easily and break the diet inadvertently, or in social circumstances where to avoid the food is difficult.

Unfortunately, there are a small number of people who, with certain foods, despite being vigilant about avoidance, are still unable to return to eating them without suffering symptoms.

Is three months exclusion too long for you?
A shorter period of avoidance will mean you will not be able to eat your problem foods very often ever again.

After one month's exclusion you may get away with eating some foods and drinks once every four days. This can be useful with, for example, cheese, wine, chocolate, but not helpful with cow's milk products, tea, coffee, or a major ingredient in bread, because most people will want or need to consume these foods every day.

If you want to be able to eat your problem food/s every day without suffering adverse symptoms, three months exclusion is essential.

Can you develop an intolerance to a new food?
Absolutely and unfortunately, yes! For anyone who has become intolerant of any food or food group, there is always the possibility you can develop new intolerances. This means your best way forward is to eat a variety of foods and not eat any one food or drink too frequently.

Frequency of use is the important key to the development of food intolerances.

Can you eat problem foods normally after three months exclusion?

Not quite. It will be sensible for you to exercise some restriction. I will be giving you hints and tips so you will not feel too hard done by read *Chapter 15: Recommended diet for your age and gender*.

Can you develop different symptoms at a later date?

Again, absolutely and unfortunately, yes!

Food intolerance symptoms can change as time passes. In the future, you may find that your problem food will give you different symptoms. This can occur commonly when there is another trigger. For more information read *Chapter 16: Appendix: Typical symptom changes in food intolerance; Common food intolerance symptoms in adults; and Common food intolerance symptoms in children*.

Case Study

Bridget came for a consultation with me when she was 58 years old. She had suffered health problems all her life. None of them had been serious but they had undoubtedly affected her quality of life.

As a bottle-fed baby in the mid 1950s, she had been very colicky and had vomited up small amounts of milk frequently. Her tummy settled down by the time she was one but she developed some eczema, which stayed with her for three or four years. When she started school she suffered from tummy aches until she was about nine years old. Between the ages of nine and twelve Bridget was afflicted by many sore throats. Her headaches began when she was 11 or 12 and she was suffering full-blown migraines by the time she was 14. When she went to university, she had her first symptoms of Irritable Bowel Syndrome, from which she has suffered ever since.

Following my recommendations, Bridget started to feel better when she avoided cow's milk products, cocoa and coffee. With the benefit of hindsight and having picked her elderly mother's brains, Bridget felt milk had been affecting her since she was a few months old.

When I explained certain triggers can change the symptoms suffered - in Bridget's case starting school, changing schools, puberty, starting university - she understood why her family and her doctors had believed the underlying cause of her symptoms had been an emotional one.

Why these foods?	Cause
Cow's milk products	Frequency of use
Cocoa	Frequency of use
Coffee	Frequency of use
Why then?	**Trigger**
Aged 5 started school	Stress
Aged 11 changed schools	Stress
Aged 11 puberty	Hormonal
Aged 18 left home for university	Stress

Read *Chapter 15: Recommended diet for your age and gender*. This chapter has been compiled using the client data that I have accumulated in my 21 years specializing in food intolerance. Before you start the exclusion diet, make sure that you read the relevant chapters for all the symptoms which you or your child suffer.

To recap

- Frequency of use is the important key to the development of food intolerances.
- If you want to be able to eat your problem foods every day without suffering adverse symptoms, three months exclusion is essential.
- Life and health stressors can trigger food intolerance to start or get worse.
- The symptoms suffered can change as time goes by.

Chapter 3: Food intolerance in children

The profile in regard to children's food intolerances is much less complicated than that for adults. The number of foods children react to is much smaller and it is uncommon for a child to react to a food or drink not frequently consumed.

The table below details the most common food intolerances from my 2015 Survey, which included 96 children of 17 years and under.

Food	Percentage
Cow's milk products	71
Orange	46
Cocoa	39
Apple	30
Sweet artificial flavours	12
Aspartame	8
Soya	2
Monosodium glutamate E621	7
E150 –E155 colour caramel	5
Sunflower	5
Wheat	>1
Honey	>1
Black grapes and raisins	>1
Blackcurrant	>1

For more information about food and additive avoidance read *Chapter 16: Appendix.*

Points to note
- Children tend to react to a more limited range of foods than adults, whatever their symptoms.
- Milk intolerance is nearly twice as likely in children as adults.

- The two children who reacted adversely to honey were rarely eating sugar. Honey was being used instead of sugar in their families. It was a frequent food for them.
- No child under 16 was intolerant of yeast. Yet yeast is a common food intolerance for many adults.
- The children who were intolerant of aspartame were drinking sugar free squashes several times every day. It was a frequent food for them.
- Children who had a problem with sweet artificial flavours were frequent sweet eaters or often drank fizzy drinks. A high percentage, 62.5% of teenagers reacted to sweet artificial flavours.
- The one child who was intolerant of wheat was on the autistic spectrum.
- One in three children were intolerant of apple, of whom 75% were under five years of age. Apple is used instead of sugar in many baby and toddler foods and drinks.
- The children for whom black grapes were a problem were both toddlers and were eating raisins several times a day. It was a frequent food for them.
- The children reacting to blackcurrant were drinking blackcurrant squashes or juice drinks several times a day. It was a frequent food for them.
- The 2% of children who reacted to soya were using several soya products daily to avoid cow's milk products. It was a frequent food for them.

Case Study

Ashok, aged eight, suffered from a painful, barking, uncontrollable cough. Asthma inhalers had no impact.

On testing, Ashok was intolerant of:

- all cow's milk products;
- fragrances in cleaning products and fabric conditioners; and
- sweet artificial flavours, found in sweets, fizzy drinks and coca cola.

Ashok liked milk, drinking approximately half a litre a day and eating cheese and yogurt daily. Ashok was allowed sweets every day after school. His regular yogurt contained sweet artificial flavours, as did the ice cream he ate for pudding every evening.

Why these foods?	Cause
Cow's milk products	Frequency of use
Sweet artificial flavours	Frequency of use
Why then?	**Trigger**
We could not work out what the trigger had been	

After one week of following my recommended exclusion diet his cough had only slightly improved, but on questioning, his mother had not managed to rid the household of all possible fragrance. Another week went by and there was still not much improvement.

However, his mum felt evenings at home were better, but he was still coughing during the school day and at weekends.

In this instance, I requested they return for some more testing and asked them to bring the actual foods Ashok regularly ate and drank. Despite the fact that Ashok's mother thought she had checked lists of ingredients well, I found his Ribena and his special "free from" biscuits contained artificial flavouring. Ribena and these biscuits were a weekend treat, hence the weekend coughing. I explained to Ashok's mum it was not necessary to use "free from" products, because there are many normal biscuits, which do not contain milk.

Unfortunately, the school coughing still continued. Eventually, I sourced a fragrance free industrial cleaning product which the school agreed to use throughout the building. This worked for Ashok immediately and he has had no coughing since!

For more information about sweet artificial flavour, read *Chapter 12: Monosodium glutamate and sweet artificial flavouring.*

Case Study

I saw Ben aged 18 months, because severe eczema was making his life really miserable. His parents were having to wet-wrap him and use steroid creams. His desire to scratch meant he often drew blood and his skin had been infected three times in the previous six months.

On testing Ben, I discovered his problem foods were:

* cow's, goat's, sheep's and buffalo milk products;
* apple; and
* fragrance in products.

As Ben was a picky eater, I suggested he take a children's multivitamin daily, and asked his mother to check apple was not used as a flavour in the vitamins she bought. I informed his mum some soya milks are sweetened with apple juice and it was necessary to read all the labels carefully. I advised her to use other milks apart from soya if possible, because of concern about feeding little boys too much soya, due to the oestrogen content.

Ben's favourite drink had always been apple juice and his mother had often given Ben Fruit Flakes as a healthy alternative to sweets. These are made of concentrated apple juice.

Why these foods?	Cause
Cow's milk products	Frequency of use
Apple	Frequency of use

I tested the products Ben's clothes were washed in and discovered he reacted to all the usual biological, non-bio products and fabric conditioners. I advised his mum to use Surcare to wash his clothes, but not to use Surcare fabric conditioner. As he had eczema in his ears, I checked his regular shampoo, Johnson's Baby Shampoo. This has a lovely fragrance and is coloured orange. Both the colour and fragrance are likely to exacerbate skin problems. I suggested the brand

Simple was used for hair washing, because this product is fragrance and colour free. I recommended they did not use soap or bubble baths.

When they came back to see me a week later, although Ben still had some patches of eczema, he had no itch and no new patches. Any new skin looked alarmingly pink. During the next two weeks his skin became smooth. His ears no longer itched. His sleep pattern had not improved but after two nights of using a controlled crying method, he was sleeping well.

Case Study

I was really concerned about Simon when I first met him. He was very pale, listless and lethargic for an eight year old. He was getting severe stomach aches about twice a week and even on the good days, he was tired and did not want to do much.

When I tested him, I was expecting, as is the case with most children who suffer with stomach symptoms that cow's milk products were at the root of the problem. However, it turned out apple and blackcurrant were the actual causes in this case. Simon's mum saw with the benefit of hindsight that the bad days were when she had apple juice in the house, a drink which Simon loved, while the better days were when they had run out of apple juice. On the better days, he drank apple and blackcurrant squash, in which the percentage of actual juice was much lower than in the 100% juice. These smaller amounts did not give him stomach ache, but did make him listless. After only two days of avoidance, Simon had no more stomach aches and he recovered his lost energy levels. I was pleased to hear from his mother, that a decision was made in the family for the children to drink more water and use a variety of fruit juices in future.

To recap
- The foods your child is reacting to are likely to be things they consume regularly three times a day or more, whatever it is, cow's milk products, a fruit or a drink, honey or aspartame.
- Cow's milk intolerance is much more common in children than adults.

Part 2: Symptoms

Chapter 4: Gastro-intestinal and digestion

It is a miserable existence for someone whose life is ruled by their gut. Pains, cramps, bloating, rushing to the toilet, all affect their quality of life.

If you are or your child are suffering from digestion symptoms, these can include; infant colic, tummy aches, bloating, wind, loose stools, diarrhoea, urgency, incontinence, constipation, indigestion, reflux, nausea and vomiting; avoiding the foods or drinks you are intolerant of will help your symptoms.

Many adults with the above symptoms are given a diagnosis of Irritable Bowel Syndrome. It sounds like a bona fide diagnosis, but means very little apart from 'your bowel is irritated by something'. If your bowel is being irritated by a food or drink, it is very likely to be one you frequently consume.

You will almost certainly have tried to work out what your problem foods are, because of symptoms suffered after certain meals. You may have decided that all kinds of things, maybe vegetables, fizzy drinks, red meat, rich meals, fibrous meals and acidic foods are aggravating your tummy.

Frequent consumption of a staple food or drink is usually the cause, but the sufferer assumes the food most recently eaten is the culprit.

The frequently consumed food upsets the gut, and then it seems anything the person eats is a problem, making them windy, bloated, giving them pain, abnormal stools, reflux or indigestion. Sufferers start to avoid anything that seems linked with the timing of their symptoms and consequently exclude an ever-increasing number of foods from their diet. Their daily menu becomes unhealthy, bland and boring, and they can end up creating new intolerances.

Even if you have a diagnosis of hiatus hernia, ulcerative colitis, colitis, diverticulitis or Crohn's disease, a change of diet can seriously improve things for you.

Case Study

Jodie, a 28 year old beauty salon owner, came to me for a food intolerance test following a recommendation from a friend. Her main problems were tummy related, but she had some other symptoms which could have been linked to food intolerance. She complained of daily bloating. This bloating was extremely uncomfortable because her tummy swelled to such an extent on some days she looked six months pregnant. Flatulence was a major problem for Jodie, particularly later in the day. Her stools were always loose and occasionally she suffered diarrhoea. When she had diarrhoea, it was preceded by pain, and associated with a very urgent need to get to the toilet. Jodie had seen her GP several times during the previous ten years. Eight years previously she had been referred for a colonoscopy, but nothing abnormal was discovered. Consequently, she had been diagnosed as suffering from Irritable Bowel Syndrome.

The other symptoms that Jodie presented with were fatigue, lethargy and joint pains in her fingers, wrists and elbows.

Jodie was suspicious of wheat, because the bloating started after lunch. She usually ate a sandwich or a wrap at lunchtime. Her diet contained very few vegetables, because she thought they were a trigger. Her GP had advised her to avoid vegetables, fizzy drinks and anything that seemed to make her more windy. I explained often with tummy issues, the person perceives that certain foods such as vegetables, spices, a rich meal, a fatty meal or a big meal can affect them. But once the underlying problem food has been excluded from the daily diet, the person can cope with the foods of which they were suspicious.

When I tested her, I discovered that Jodie was intolerant of:

- cow's milk products; and
- dark brown food colouring E150-E155.

Jodie used cow's milk on cereal every morning, in two cups of tea and two cups of coffee daily. She ate cheese most days, and ate at least one yogurt a day. I explained to Jodie that people become intolerant of foods they tend to eat or drink most frequently. She quickly realised that cow's milk products were the food group that she consumed more often than any other food or drink, on average seven to eight times daily.

Dark brown food colour is in cola drinks, gravy and stock cubes mainly. Jodie had noticed that she felt even worse after a roast dinner, but thought it was because it was a large meal, or because the vegetables had made her windy. When she felt worse after a diet coke, she presumed that it was because of the bubbles.

Why these foods?	Cause
Cow's milk products	Frequency of use
Why then?	**Trigger**
Starts the pill age 20 [symptoms started]	Hormonal
Recent work stress [symptoms worsened]	Stress

Jodie agreed to avoid these foods, and after a week she was feeling much better. She suffered a few headaches in the first few days because of withdrawal symptoms, but her tummy settled down. She had much more energy and was no longer lethargic. Her joint pains completely disappeared. The only hiccough she encountered was when she ate goat's cheese. Her tummy became very bloated again. She assumed, following an email conversation with me, that she could not tolerate any animal milks, cheeses or yogurts.

After three months exclusion, Jodie gradually reintroduced her problem foods. Now she eats cow's products again, but tries not to have them more than twice a day. She has learned to enjoy her coffee black, and uses almond milk in her tea and coconut milk on her cereal. When Jodie introduced E150 [caramel] in the form of coca cola again, she felt bloated within four hours and was back to feeling unaccountably tired. Instead she has lemonade if she wants to have a fizzy drink. She has learned to make her own gravy using marmite instead of gravy granules.

The table below details the most common food intolerances of the 345 adults and 96 children who suffered tummy symptoms in my 2015 Survey.

Food	Percentage of adults	Percentage of children
Milk	37	82
Cocoa	41	46
Coffee	33	0
Orange	31	50
Yeast, cheese, yogurt	38	0
Tea	29	0
Some form of alcohol	11	n/a
Sweet artificial flavours	15	20
Apple	11	31
Monosodium glutamate	9	10
E150 [caramel] dark brown food colour	14	7
Aspartame	3	11
Soya	3	10
Sunflower	7	5
Wheat	>1	0

Points to note

- In children with tummy symptoms, cow's milk products are a cause in 11% more cases than for all other symptoms.
- Orange intolerance in children with tummy symptoms is 4% higher than for other symptoms.
- In adults, coffee is 4% more likely to be a cause of tummy problems, than it is for all other symptoms, whereas tea remains the same.
- More children with tummy symptoms, 20%, react adversely to sweet artificial flavours compared to 12% of children with other symptoms.

Case Study

Louise a lawyer aged 31, came to see me for testing because she had major problems with constipation, wind and abdominal pain. She occasionally had loose stools and on those days had a real problem, needing to find a toilet fast, sometimes so urgently that she felt uneasy about leaving the house on a bad day. Also, she was suffering from frequent headaches. She felt unaccountably tired. Louise felt that her GP was 'losing the will to live' every time she pitched up at the surgery. Louise told me that until three years before, she was really healthy apart from suffering from acne. She had been put on the pill to help her severe acne and although her skin was now clear, she had never felt well since. Her tummy issues and headaches had started within one month of taking the pill.

At around the same time she had suffered a very painful split from a long term boyfriend. Her GP's approach mainly consisted of saying that Louise was suffering from stress and would be helped by being able to relax more. Louise recognised that her job was a stressor, she worked long hours and she was anxious, but she felt that her anxiety was because of her health concerns and not vice versa.

Louise thought that bread might be a part of her constipation problems, but, like many other people, she felt that it was from the wheat component. Despite having avoided wheat for a while, she recognised this was not the full story.

On testing, I found Louise was intolerant of:

- yeast, all cheeses and all yogurts;
- coffee; and
- cocoa.

Louise loved cheese! Also, she regularly ate yogurt. By cutting out wheat, she had mostly cut out yeast, because she did not like the taste of wheat or gluten free breads. But, she was still eating cheese daily. Because Louise was so tired, she had got into the habit of using coffee to keep herself awake. She was therefore having up to six or seven strong coffees daily. She said she rarely ate chocolate and could not understand why she had become intolerant of cocoa. I explained to her that the coffee bean and cocoa bean are very close relatives. When one of them is a major problem the other can give similar symptoms. Of interest to me was the fact that Louise had felt extremely well when on holiday in Thailand. While there, she hardly drunk any coffee and rarely ate bread or cheese. By taking my advice and avoiding these foods in her diet, Louise was headache ad tummy symptom free within 11 days.

She was far more energetic and her fatigue was minimal despite her job being demanding and stressful. I had suggested to her that she reduce her coffee intake by one mug a day during one week, so her withdrawal symptoms were not too severe.

I felt the trigger for Louise to start suffering from food intolerances had been starting the pill. She was not happy about being on it anyway, so decided to stop. Her one concern with regard to stopping the pill, though, was that her acne might return. I told her that one of the commonest food intolerance causes of acne is cheese, so I felt fairly confident that if she followed my suggested diet her severe acne would not return even if she stopped taking the pill.

Why those foods?	Cause
Coffee	Frequency of use
Cocoa	Too close to coffee
Yeast, cheese, yogurt	Frequency of use
Why then?	**Trigger**
Starting the pill	Hormonal
Relationship break-up	Stress
Stressful job	Stress
Health anxiety	Stress

On testing Louise for vitamin and mineral deficiencies, I found she was Vitamin A deficient. One of the symptoms of Vitamin A deficiency is adult acne. I suggested she take Vitamin A in the form of Beta-carotene 15mg, which she agreed to do. Louise's acne did not return when she stopped the pill. Louise chose not to introduce most of her problem foods back into her regular diet, because she felt so much better and did not want to risk feeling unwell again. She did miss cheese and maybe eats it once a fortnight. Because she likes wraps, she is using those instead of bread.

Case Study

Caitlin was 11 when I first met her. She had missed on average three days a week schooling in the previous term. Every day, all day, she felt sick. Her tummy was always uncomfortable and frequently very painful, on which occasions she suffered acute diarrhoea. On really bad days she felt too unwell to attend school. Also, she was extremely tired.

Poor Caitlin was very pale and lethargic on the day that I tested her. She had a history of loose stools as a baby, which had responded well to a change from a cow's milk formula to one with a soya base.

She had suffered with eczema as a toddler. The eczema stopped when she was around six years old when she started getting tummy symptoms again. Her parents reduced the amount of dairy products that she was consuming, with good effect.

Six months before I saw her Caitlin had moved to high school and had found the transition hard. Within a few weeks at the new school, her tummy symptoms had started again.

The school felt the problem was an emotional one. She was seen by a paediatrician who suggested a gluten free diet and that she use lactofree products. This made minimal improvement to her distressing symptoms and child psychiatry was being considered, when Caitlin's mother found my website and requested an appointment.

On testing, I discovered Caitlin was intolerant of:

- cow's milk products;
- E471 and E472;
- apple; and
- cocoa.

Lactofree products will not help people who are intolerant of all cow's milk products. The people for whom these products are suitable are those who do not produce enough lactase enzyme in their small intestine, and as a consequence cannot digest lactose [milk sugar]. Lactofree milk is normal milk with lactase added, so for Caitlin the use of lactofree milk made no difference to her symptoms. E471 and E472, Mono and Diglycerides of fatty acids, are emulsifiers which are found in many breads and margarines. Caitlin may have seen some improvement in her symptoms when she was using the gluten free bread, because it did not contain those emulsifiers, whereas the family's preferred brand did.

Caitlin loved apple juice, drank it two or three times a day and ate an apple most days.

Caitlin used to eat chocolate every day, but thought that it made her more nauseous. She had stopped eating it four weeks or so before she saw me.

Luckily for Caitlin she was better within three days of changing her diet to my recommendations. Child psychiatry was not necessary, and she is enjoying school now that she feels well.

Why those foods?	Cause
Cow's milk products	Frequency of use
Orange	Past frequency of use
Why then?	Trigger
Starting high school	Stress

Case Study

Barbara aged 53, had been suffering for 18 months from Irritable Bowel symptoms, including enormous amounts of embarrassing wind and almost daily bloating. She occasionally suffered loose stools and on those days, not to put too fine a point on it, would often let go a 'wet fart'. Otherwise, she tended to be pretty constipated and only opened her bowels twice a week.

Movicol had been little help with any of her symptoms. Colonoscopy had been performed a few months before Barbara came to see me, but the results had been normal.

Barbara also suffered from an extremely irritating rash on her neck and torso.

On testing, I found Barbara was intolerant of:

- all tea, including green tea and redbush tea; and
- fragrances in products.

Barbara's regular tea intake was high, up to eight a day on a weekday, when she drank it regularly in the office.

Fragrances in products were aggravating Barbara's skin rash, and she reacted adversely to her regular Persil non-bio and Comfort 'Pure' fabric conditioner. I advised Barbara to use the brand Surcare to wash her clothes, but not to use the Surcare fabric conditioner at all. She loved Radox bath and shower products, but I explained that these, being so highly perfumed and coloured were also affecting her rash. She agreed to try Simple products. Her normal shampoos were also a problem and because the itchy rash was present on her back and neck, she agreed to try Simple shampoo and conditioner.

Two or three weeks later, Barbara emailed me to say she had seen little improvement in her symptoms. So we arranged an appointment for further testing. On questioning, Barbara said she had been quite hopeful as, although she had quite a bad headache in the first few days of following the recommended diet her tummy had been much more comfortable and her skin less itchy.

However, after a couple of days, it had all worsened again. On testing we found she had started to react to coffee. Following my advice, she was only having two coffees daily. Therefore, I wondered why she had been so unlucky. It turned out that a few years previously, Barbara had been a big coffee drinker and following a bout of flu, had gone off coffee in a big way, leading to complete avoidance. She still did not like the drink very much, but felt almost forced to join in the office tea/coffee drinking system. I think what happened was very quickly, she developed a new intolerance. Sometimes our bodies are trying to tell us something if we 'go off' a previously favoured food or drink.

Why those foods?	Cause
Tea	Frequency of use
Green tea, redbush tea	Too close to normal tea
Coffee	Aversion and former frequency of use
Why then?	**Trigger**
Menopause	Hormonal

In addition to my suggested change of diet, if you do not see a marked improvement, there are some basic self-help actions you can take to enable your gastro-intestinal tract to function better. I know many of you will have tried these things because they are very obvious suggestions, but if you have not, it may help.

- Sit up straight when eating. Digestive organs have no room to function well if you are slumped.
- Never eat with your mouth open, air gets in!
- Eat slowly, one mouthful at a time, well chewed. Put your utensils down while chewing, so you are not tempted to eat so fast.

Supplements to take if you still have symptoms despite a change of diet.

Take these supplements for at least a month.

- Polyzyme Forte from Biocare, which contains digestive enzymes and probiotics. Initially you will need to take this with every meal.
- L Glutamine powder 5g at night. L Glutamine helps to heal the gut.

Should you not see any improvement following a change of diet and taking these supplements, you will find it helpful to consult a nutritionist. Make sure that the person is BANT [British Association of Nutritional Therapists] registered.

Still no change?

Consult your GP.

To recap
- Gastro-intestinal symptoms will be triggered by frequent daily foods or drinks.
- Lactofree products are not milk free.
- Probiotics and gastric enzymes can help those whose symptoms do not completely go away with a change of diet.

Chapter 5: Headache and migraine

At best, sufferers have occasional headaches that make them feel under par, but able to cope with what life throws at them. At worst, a full-blown migraine can catapult a sufferer into a maelstrom of extreme headache, appalling nausea, scary sensations in their arms, visual disturbance, and an awareness that they have to go to bed and exclude all day and artificial light. I have been aware for a long time there is not just one reason for a migraine starting, but a combination of several causes. All causes need to be considered to achieve the best possible outcome for the headache and migraine sufferer.

My 2015 Survey consisted of 345 adults, including 109 suffering headache and 52 migraine. The foods, products and vitamin and mineral deficiencies, which were the most common causes are tabled below. I only included people who suffered frequent or daily headaches, rather than those who occasionally had a mild headache.

Cause	Percentages of adult headache sufferers	Percentages of adult migraine sufferers
Chemical fragrance	62	75
Cow's milk products	42	42
Vitamin B6 deficiency	40	76
Cocoa	44	42
Yeast, cheeses, yogurts	36	37
Coffee	32	33
Chromium deficiency	24	62
Tea	24	26
Orange	24	26
Sweet artificial flavours	17	9

Points to note

Comparing these figures with those for adults suffering IBS symptoms, there are several marked differences.

- Vitamin B6 deficiency is common in headache and migraine sufferers, with 40% of headache sufferers and 76% of migraine sufferers, compared with 25% of people with IBS.
- Chromium deficiency is more common, with 24% of people suffering from headaches and 62% of people suffering from migraines, compared to 11% of IBS sufferers.
- Chemical fragrances in the environment in the form of air fresheners, fragranced candles, incense sticks and fabric conditioners, are commonly linked with headache and migraine symptoms. 62% of those with headaches and 75% of those with migraines.

The table below details the results from the same 2015 Survey for 22 children with headache and migraine symptoms.

Cause	Percentage of children with headache and migraine
Cow's milk products	95
Fragrances	62
	100 of migraine sufferers
Cocoa	50
Orange	41
Apple	24
Vitamin B6 deficiency	24
Sweet artificial flavours	19

Points to note

- The percentage of cow's milk intolerance is much higher than for any other symptom.
- Fragrances feature in two thirds of children with headaches and in all migraine sufferers
- Cocoa was only a problem if the child was consuming something chocolate-flavoured daily.

During my 21 years of food intolerance experience, I have expanded my knowledge to provide the most informed advice I can. One important observation I want to share with you is; people only get the best results if they follow all the advice provided. Do not cherry pick the aspects that appeal most or are easiest for you to follow, and disregard the rest. Do everything I suggest right from the start. The food/drink/product you feel you cannot give up is likely to be the worst thing for you.

Case Study

Sean, aged ten, was missing a lot of school because of his headaches. They affected him nearly every day. The result was a young man who was not getting much fun out of life. His parents had separated at around the time that the headaches began and many people felt there was an emotional cause. His GP focussed on reassuring Sean all would be well.

On testing, I found that Sean was intolerant of:

- cow's milk products;
- blackcurrant; and
- chemical fragrance.

Sean ate cow's milk products four times a day or more. I explained to him and his mother the reason milk was a problem was because it was the most frequent food he had every day. Blackcurrant, in the form of Ribena, was the next most common item in his daily intake. I recommended he drink more water and only use other flavours of fruit squash once, or a maximum of twice daily.

Why those foods?	Cause
Cow's milk products	Frequency of use
Blackcurrant	Frequency of use
Why then?	**Trigger**
Influenza virus	Illness

On my advice, the family stopped using fabric conditioners, boxed up their fragranced candles and used fragrance free cleaning sprays and polishes.

Within three days, Sam was headache free.

Other causes of headache:
- high blood pressure;
- problems with eyesight;
- out of date spectacle prescription;
- dehydration; drink a glass of water when you have the beginnings of a headache, to see if that will help;
- tooth grinding can cause headaches; see your dentist;
- neck, and shoulder stiffness, tension and pain can lead to headaches; see a physiotherapist, osteopath or chiropractor.

Blood sugar control and chromium deficiency
If someone is deficient in the mineral chromium, they will often suffer headaches and migraines when their blood sugar levels are low. The chromium deficient person will already know he/she needs to eat frequently or is likely to suffer the following symptoms:

- headache;
- irritability;
- nausea;
- shaky feelings; and
- sugar craving.

For many of these people, the underlying cause is a chromium deficiency and there it is, seventh on the adult list of causes of headaches and third for migraines. Chromium is the mineral responsible for the regulation of blood sugar levels.

Solutions if you suspect you have a problem regulating your blood sugar levels.

- Eat frequently, every few hours, rather than having big meals and large gaps in between.
- Avoid sugar fixing, which is something you have found helps your symptoms. You eat something sweet, [often chocolate] and feel better, with the headache, nausea, irritability and shakiness all gone fast! Eating something sweet raises the blood sugar quickly, which leads the body to overcompensate and produce insulin. This has the effect of sending blood sugar plummeting down. The whole cycle starts again with irritability, shaking, sugar craving, nausea and headache. You eat something sugary again to feel better, which means more insulin production and your blood sugar drops again.
- Eat more complex carbohydrate, e.g. brown or wholemeal grains in bread, ryevita and rice cakes. These keep your blood sugar at a moderate level for longer periods of time than sugar and refined [white] carbohydrates.
- Eat more protein. Energy from protein this kicks in when the energy from the carbohydrate runs out, and is useful if you come to a low ebb at mid-morning or mid-afternoon. It is helpful for blood sugar levels to eat protein for breakfast, e.g. an egg, or bacon, and to eat more protein at lunchtime. Nuts are a good healthy snack to have in your desk drawer.

The foods that reduce chromium absorption are:
- sugar:
- refined foods; and
- alcohol.

Here is another vicious circle. Eat too much sugar and you reduce chromium absorption. If you have symptoms which are suggestive of problems with blood sugar control, take a chromium supplement, 200-400mg depending on your size and weight. This helps to reduce sugar craving and keeps your blood sugar more stable. It is still important to eat in a way that stops your blood sugar shooting up and down.

The diet which helps those with a blood sugar regulation problem is the GL [Glycaemic Load] diet. There are many books written about this and it will benefit you to learn more.

For more information about chromium deficiency read *Chapter 16: Appendix.*

Chemical fragrance

Breathing in artificial fragrance can affect people in many different ways. I have found with headaches and migraines, that fragrances in the environment are a massive part of the cause.

Since I have been testing products with added fragrance and suggesting clients avoid using them, my percentage improvements for headache and migraine, have risen from 70% average improvement in 2003 to 95% + average improvement in 2015. Stop using fabric conditioners, air fresheners, plug-in air fresheners, incense sticks, fragranced diffusers, body butters, polish and spray cleaners with added fragrance. For more information read *Chapter 16: Appendix.*

These types of products are a big aggravation for headache and migraine sufferers. Remove them from your home. It is important and will help you feel better.

Over use of painkillers

Many painkillers are addictive when used a few times daily for a few weeks. A person who is addicted to painkillers will get a headache when they need another dose of the painkiller to which they have become addicted. Stopping the painkillers is a difficult process, because of the severe withdrawal symptoms that are bound to result. The headaches should clear within a week or so.

Case Study

Sandy aged 47, came to see me because she was suffering headaches four or five times a week. She suffered a migraine on average twice a month. Her migraine would always announce itself with an aura, which she described as an awareness that something was about to 'kick off'. She experienced a vague flashing light experience and she knew if she did not take her Fexofenadine within five minutes she would be in deep trouble. If the migraine were to develop into a bad one, she knew she would need to go to bed for at least 24 hours. Sandy would suffer severe nausea and need to stay in a darkened room for the duration of the migraine. She had a son, aged 13 with a severe learning disability and very challenging behaviour. Sandy found it impossible to manage him when her migraine hit. This was becoming increasingly problematic for her husband to come home early from work.

On first meeting Sandy, it was evident to me she was trying hard to cope. She was leading a life overloaded with stress. She had no leisure time. She hated having to ask people for help. Sandy loved her son, but he was very difficult to manage. She was living on a knife-edge. Sandy was also suffering other symptoms including mood swings, irritability and mild depression. She struggled to get a good night's sleep and was waking up in the night desperate for something sweet to eat. She would then eat several Weight Watchers chocolate biscuits. This would calm her and she could sleep again. When I explained to her about blood sugar levels and the link with the symptoms she was suffering, it suddenly made sense. She had gained a lot of weight during the previous year and joined Weight Watchers. However, in following the Weight Watchers diet she had reduced her protein intake because meat is particularly heavy on calories. She had started eating low fat yogurt even though she did not enjoy it and she was using many Weight Watchers products. This meant she was homing in increasingly on chocolate bars, biscuits and cakes.

On testing, I found Sandy was reacting adversely to:

- cow's milk products;
- cocoa;
- chemical fragrances; and
- most white wines.

Why those foods?	Cause
Cow's milk products	Frequency of use
Cocoa	Frequency of use
White wine	Frequency of use
Why then?	**Trigger**
Disabled son	Stress
Depression	Stress

Sandy was deficient in:

- vitamin B6; and
- chromium.

I advised her to take a vitamin B complex containing between 80mg and 100mg of vitamin B6, and to choose a milk free supplement. I suggested she take 400mg of milk free chromium. Sandy stopped eating milk, cocoa and drinking white wines, having a drink of vodka sometimes instead.

Within nine days, she was feeling much better. She tried eating Halloumi, a sheep's milk cheese, but felt irritable and had a headache within a few hours. It turned out that her version of Halloumi was a combination of cow's and sheep's cheese, but just in case, we did a quick retest to see whether she could tolerate sheep's products. Unfortunately, sheep's and goat's cheeses were not suitable either, so I advised Sandy to avoid all animal milk products.

She changed her cleaning products to fragrance free.

She no longer has plug-in air fresheners in the house, nor in her car. Fabric conditioners are a thing of the past.

It is early days for Sandy. At the time of writing, she has been following my advice completely for Two months. Hopefully, she will be able to reintroduce foods soon without ill effects. I informed her fragrance might be a long term problem for her, but she is not intending to use those products again. One very positive outcome is that Sandy lost a stone in weight and is feeling so much better in herself.

She has found the confidence to look for and be accepted for a part time job in a local school. She has felt better enough to get back in touch with old friends and is enjoying herself.

Case Study
The last time I saw Lewis he was 24. I had tested him three times before when he was 14, 19 and 22 years old. On each occasion he was suffering from headaches and migraines.

At the age of 14, his food intolerances were:

- cow's milk products; and
- cocoa.

He followed the advice I gave him and avoided these foods strictly for three months, after which he had tried to eat those foods in moderation.

At the age of 19, he was in his first year at university and as a young student, was burning the candle at both ends and eating rubbish food. He was using energy drinks and ProPlus [paracetamol with added caffeine] to enable him to keep awake in the daytime because he was struggling with his sleep pattern at night.

On testing Lewis, I discovered he was reacting adversely to:

- caffeine, in the ProPlus tablets and energy drink; and
- sweet artificial flavours, in the energy drinks and multitude of sweets and fizzy drinks he was using.

Lewis had a really hard time removing those foods from his diet because they are massively addictive, but he managed it, albeit over the course of two weeks. Four days after his last energy drink, he felt better. His mind was clear, he had no headache and he felt more able to concentrate on his studies again. His sleep pattern was better on weekdays but still went haywire at weekends.

When I next met Lewis he was 22. He had been feeling really well for several years, but had started to suffer from migraines again in the previous month. This coincided with his starting an unpaid internship in the finance district of the City of London. It involved a complicated commute and Lewis was out of the house for 11 hours every weekday. He was feeling exhausted and struggling to hold it all together and as a result, he was suffering.

On testing Lewis a third time, I discovered he reacted to:

- cocoa;
- E471 mono and diglycerides of fatty acids; and
- chemical fragrance.

He was deficient in:

- vitamin B6; and
- chromium.

Lewis was eating chocolate because he did not have long for lunch and it gave him a bit of a pick-up when he was feeling exhausted. E471 is an emulsifier, which is in many but not all bread, baked goods and margarines. He was eating bread containing this emulsifier two or three times a day, and it was in his favoured margarine.

His mother was keen on using plug-in air fresheners since the family had bought a dog. These fragrances are a major irritant for headache and migraine sufferers.

Within four days of following my advice he was headache free. He decided to routinely take vitamin B6 and chromium because he felt those supplements were a big support for his headaches. Also, he found it easier not to eat chocolate and sweet things when he was taking the chromium supplement.

Why those foods?	Cause
On all occasions and for all of the foods	Frequency of use
Why then?	**Trigger**
At age 14 puberty	Hormonal
At age 19 leaving home for university	Stress
At age 22 long commute and new job	Stress

The fourth time that I met Lewis he was 24 years old. He had been suffering severe migraines for the previous four months. On testing, I found that there were no food intolerances. In an attempt to reduce the severity of the migraines, and therefore be able to manage a working day, he had been taking Sumatriptan tablets several times a day. This drug should not be taken more than twice a week. Lewis had become addicted. Whenever the level of the drug in his blood dropped his headache came on. When he had a 'fix' of Sumatriptan the headache was temporarily relieved. I advised Lewis to stop using Sumatriptan as soon as possible, and warned he was likely to have severe headaches for a week or so as his addiction waned. Lewis decided to take a week off work while he was going through the withdrawal symptoms. A week later he was headache and migraine free.

To recap

- Vitamin B6 and chromium deficiencies are common in headache and migraine. It will help to take a supplement.
- For all headache and migraine sufferers, rid your home, car and if possible your workplace, of chemical fragrances [read *Chapter 16: Appendix*].
- If you are taking painkillers every day, it may be that addiction to them is the cause of your headache or migraine.

Chapter 6: Skin conditions and adult acne

The visibility of skin conditions, and the embarrassment that sufferers can feel because of the way they look, is very hard to live with. Add to that the incessant itch that an eczema sufferer has to deal with day to day, and it makes living with a chronic skin condition a miserable process. There are several factors, which when combined, can cause or aggravate a skin condition. These include:

- food intolerance;
- chemicals in products used for washing clothes, in shower gels and soaps;
- zinc deficiency; and
- stress.

Food intolerance

The usual rules apply with regard to which foods are likely to lead to an intolerant reaction, frequently consumed foods or drinks, with the sufferer consuming them more than twice a day. As with other symptoms, there are fewer foods that affect children compared to adults. Please see charts below.

This is the chart of results for adults, with percentages for each food, deficiency or fragrance related to various skin conditions for 113 adults in my 2015 Survey.

Causes	Percentage of adults	Percentage of adults	Percentage of adults	Percentage of adults	Percentage of adults
	Eczema	Rash	Itch	Acne	Urticaria
Chemical fragrance	100	70	94	40	50
Zinc deficiency	87	89	94	51	42
Cow's milk products	61	62	47	29	25

Cocoa	43	53	44	38	33
Orange	39	41	39	25	8
Coffee	48	41	44	25	33
Yeast, cheese, yogurt	30	35	28	46	17
Tea	35	29	33	38	33
Sweet artificial flavours	13	12	6	8	8
Apple	22	12	16	4	0
Vitamin A deficiency	0	24	0	63	0

These were the percentages for 40 children with eczema from my 2015 Survey.

Cause	Percentage
Fragrances	95
Cow's milk products	88
Orange	55
Zinc deficiency	38
Cocoa	33
Apple	33
Sweet artificial flavours	20
Monosodium glutamate	10

Points to note

- Although chemical fragrances in products feature at the top of both lists for eczema sufferers, with 95% of all adults and children, intolerances to foods were always part of the picture.
- With adults and children, those presenting with itch alone [with no rash] were far more likely to be caused by products e.g. those used in clothes washing, soaps, bubble baths and shower gels, rather than food. I have anecdotal evidence from clients who changed their diet, with no apparent improvement in itch, and who

subsequently changed soap, clothes washing products and bubble baths, and stopped itching.

- Acne was not often associated with adverse reactions to products, unless the person had noticed their face felt sore or tight after washing their hair, or had suffered any kind of skin reaction with cosmetics. The fragrance and colour in shampoo, soap or cosmetics was otherwise not linked with the acne.
- Chemical fragrance was closely linked with eczema and itch, and with rashes less commonly, especially if the rash was urticaria or hives. In cases of urticaria or hives food was the sole cause.
- A higher percentage of children with eczema had a cow's milk intolerance, with 88% compared to 78% of all the children in the study. In adults a similar pattern was observed, with 61% compared to 38%.
- Comparing the skin charts with my results charts for adults and children, the results were very similar in relation to sweet artificial flavours found in fizzy drinks and sweets. Those who ate or drank these products most days were likely to have become intolerant of them, including 62.5% of teenagers with skin conditions.

When you are trying to sort out your skin follow all my recommendations below:
- food intolerance diet for your age and gender;
- zinc supplementation;
- avoid products with fragrances and colours; and
- reduce stress if you recognise this as a major problem for you.

Cherry picking the ones that seem easiest just does not work. You need to do it all.

Fragrance and colour in products
As you can see from the charts above a large percentage of people with skin conditions react to fragrances and colours in the products they use.

If the skin condition affects any part of your body you will need to change the products you use to wash your clothes, and soaps, bubble baths and shower gels.

If the skin condition is on your face or scalp you will need to change shampoos and conditioners.

If the condition affects your hands, you will need to change shampoos, conditioners, soaps, shower gels and washing up liquids.

Some people's skin will cope with non-biological clothes washing products. But others will not. Better safe than sorry...change to using the brand Surcare. Do not use Surcare fabric conditioner, because it makes some people itch.

Ensure that any shampoo, soap, shower gel, bubble bath or washing up liquid is fragrance and colour free. For nearly everyone a change to the brand Simple is a good option. Surcare do a washing up liquid, or you could wear cotton lined rubber gloves or vinyl gloves.

For a very small proportion of people the brand Simple is unsuitable. If this is the case for you, source an all 'natural' product, but ensure that it is clear or white in colour, and is naturally fragranced.

Zinc deficiency
The mineral zinc is essential for healthy skin, and a deficiency will nearly always result in the person having some problems with the skin.

For more information read *Chapter 16: Appendix.*

Stress
Life stresses may be playing a part in your skin condition, but unless you are very stressed and/or anxious, following the points above usually sorts out peoples' skin problems. If you know you are stressed and anxious, deal with it by:
- getting help with your workload;
- reducing working hours;
- changing your job;
- taking time out to relax;
- hypnotherapy;

- relaxation tapes or techniques;
- yoga;
- having more fun; and
- getting counselling, psychotherapy or life coaching.

Acne

When an adult suffers acne, there can be several causes, including:

- food intolerance is likely to be a major cause and you can follow the diet I recommend for you in *Chapter 15: Suggested diets for your age and gender*;
- certain vitamin and mineral deficiencies can pre-dispose to acne; and
- occasionally, the products you use on your skin can aggravate acne.

It is not common for skin products to be the cause of acne, but sometimes acne sufferers find this to be the case. If you have noticed that the skin on your face is made sore, tight, red or overdry by proprietary acne treatments, creams and lotions, please avoid them. The chemicals in these products are mainly aimed at reducing grease and can be very strong. If you are not a teenager and you use these products, you are likely to find your skin will be sore, red and overdry.

You may experience the same problem with certain shampoos, soaps and face washes. The culprits in these products are most often colour and fragrance. If your face feels tight, dry and sore after washing your hair, try the brand Simple, which has no colour or fragrance to it. This brand provides soaps, shampoos, cleansing wipes, face washes, moisturisers and sun cream. They are suitable for most people, but occasionally they can cause an adverse reaction. If that is the case for you, source a product with natural fragrance and no added colour.

Vitamin A deficiency

According to my data, a large majority of my clients with adult acne are deficient in vitamin A. A safe and sensible way to take vitamin A is in the form of Beta-carotene. Vitamin A in too high a dose can cause liver damage. Please take 15mg Beta-carotene daily and ensure the tablet is milk and yeast free. Roaccutane, which you may have been prescribed previously, is a form of vitamin A.

Zinc deficiency

This is very commonly associated with acne. For more information read *Chapter 16: Appendix.*

Case Study

Beth was a student nurse in Cardiff, who had completed her first year and really felt she had found her ideal job. She was not especially enthusiastic about her study or lecture time in university, but was loving her practical sessions in the classroom and although she was lacking confidence on the wards, she knew this was the job for her. Unfortunately her eczema, which had not troubled her since she was a toddler, began to affect her again. As it had been when she was little, the eczema appeared behind her knees and in the creases of her elbows. Also, it was on her face, which was affecting her confidence with people. But the worst thing for her was that her hands were in a terrible state, where the eczema was always visible and quite frequently infected. Despite the judicious use of steroid creams and topical antibiotic and anti-fungal creams when necessary, there was little improvement and the probability was that she would have to give up nursing.

On testing Beth, I found her problem foods were:

- cow's milk products;
- green tea; and
- cocoa.

She was reacting adversely to fragrances in products and she was deficient in the mineral zinc.

Beth loved cheese and chocolate, and but because she was a bit overweight, she did not want to eat them every day. Instead she ate low fat cottage cheese three or four times a week and allowed herself a pizza at the weekends. Chocolate was a battle for her too, but she still ate it several times a week.

Beth had decided to eat low fat yogurt a couple of times a day, as she felt it was good for her. She knew that since she had left home she had not been eating as healthily as she used to. Following research on the internet into eczema, she had been drinking a lot of green tea, six mugs a day!

Why these foods?	Cause
Cow's milk products	Frequency of use
Green tea	Frequency of use
Why then?	**Trigger**
Starting university	Stress

I tested her regular shampoos and shower gels, and the soap and washing up liquid she used at home, and found that all products with fragrances were a problem for her. I explained that any product with fragrance or any colour other than white or clear was likely to aggravate her skin wherever it touched it. I recommended that she change her shampoo, soap, shower gel, washing up liquid and clothes washing products. I suggested she switch to the brand Simple for soap, hand wash, shower gel and shampoo, and the brand Surcare, for clothes washing and washing up liquid. I suggested Beth use vinyl gloves when washing up or hair washing, but once her hands healed, she found this was not necessary.

There was a problem regarding the anti-bacterial hand wash used in hospital, but she was given special permission to use Simple hand wash when in the nursing school practising.

She still had to use the recommended hand wash on the hospital wards. Luckily, by the time she had her next ward placement, her hand eczema was much better and her skin seemed to cope with using a stronger product. The eczema on her face, knees and elbows disappeared when she avoided her problem foods, drinks, and products and when she was taking 30mg of zinc daily.

Case Study

Shanelle, aged 22, had been suffering from an unbearable itch for two and a half years. There was no visible rash but sometimes her scalp itched. Very often her ears were driving her mad, to the extent that she wanted to relieve the itch by poking inside them with anything she could find. Her body was rarely itch free and was always worse after a shower. Shanelle had tried lukewarm showers, but it had not made any difference. Shanelle also had symptoms of Irritable Bowel Syndrome, with bloating and loose stools, which she had suffered since she had been extremely unwell with the Norovirus.

On testing Shanelle, I found she was intolerant of:

- cocoa;
- coffee; and
- artificial fragrance.

Why these foods?	Cause
Cow's milk products	Frequency of use
Green tea	Frequency of use
Why then?	Trigger
Starting university	Stress

The itch was the worst symptom for Shanelle. Because of this I asked her to change her clothes washing products to Surcare, using no fabric conditioner in the first instance, and change all her hair and body washing products to the brand Simple, before changing her diet. By making these changes she reported that her itch was gone everywhere except for her ears. I advised her to see her GP about this and the itch went when she had used a steroid based ear spray for a week. When she tried a fragranced shampoo two months later, the itch in her ears returned immediately.

Shanelle's skin did improve on a change of diet, but her stomach was not completely better until she took some digestive enzymes and probiotic supplements.

Case Study

Polina, a charming 31 year old, hailed from a small town in Poland. She was suffering severe acne. She had been prescribed the pill for many years to help the condition and it had worked well for Polina. But she had plans to start a family and therefore had stopped using oral contraception. This resulted in her acne returning really badly. Poor Polina was really embarrassed about her skin, and was feeling really low.

On testing, the only food she was reacting to was cheese. Polina loved cheese of any sort. She wondered whether she might get away with using sheep's or goat's cheeses. But when cheese alone is a problem for someone, it encompasses all cheeses, even vegan, not just cow's cheeses.

I discovered that Polina was deficient in:

- vitamin A; and
- zinc.

I recommended she take Beta-carotene 15mg and zinc 30mg daily.

After ten days, when Polina's skin was improving but not completely better, I offered, as is always the case, to do more testing at no extra charge. On retesting, she had developed a problem with cocoa.

I had tested cocoa ten days earlier and there was no problem, but Polina explained that she had a suspicion that chocolate made her spots worse and so had not been using it for a month or so. On being told that all was well she had, during that ten days, been enjoying her favourite snack. She was using cocoa daily, and had redeveloped the old intolerance.

Why those foods?	Cause
Cheese	Frequency of use
Cocoa	Frequency of use
Why then?	**Trigger**
Stopping the contraceptive pill	Hormonal

Five days later without chocolate, she had lovely clear skin.

To recap

- With nearly all skin conditions food intolerance is the main cause.
- When there is an itch without a rash, the cause is often the use of products, which are coloured or fragranced. Food might not be implicated.
- Zinc supplementation helps all skin conditions.
- Using products that are fragrance and colour free helps all skin conditions.
- Beta-carotene supplementation helps acne sufferers.

Chapter 7: Asthma, catarrh, cough and rhinitis

Symptoms that affect noses, throats and lungs such as rhinitis, catarrh, post-nasal drip, recurrent sore throats, catarrh, cough, throat clearing, glue ear and asthma are usually caused by a combination of factors, including:

- food intolerance;
- natural substances in the environment the sufferer is exposed to, for example pollens, house dust mite, mould spores, feathers and cigarette smoke; and
- man made products the sufferer is exposed to, e.g. cleaning products, cheap fragrances, petrol, diesel and gloss paint.

Most people who suffer from asthma, catarrh and rhinitis have been prescribed steroid inhalers and nasal sprays. These work well for many, but can sometimes lose their effectiveness with prolonged use.

The following table details the results from my 2015 Survey, which included 345 adults and 96 children, of which 132 were asthma, catarrh, rhinitis, chronic cough or throat clearing sufferers.

Cause	Percentage
Food intolerance	100
Chemical fragrance	79
Feathers	62
Mould	15
Tree grass flower pollens	13
Gloss paint	10
Cigarette smoke	5
House dust mite	2
Petrol and diesel	>1

Points to note

- All asthma, catarrh and rhinitis sufferers were intolerant of some foods or drinks.
- Those who reacted to mould were aware they had a damp problem in their home.
- The adults who reacted to cigarette smoke, either hated the smell or knew it affected their breathing. Without exception, the children whose symptoms were exacerbated by cigarette smoke had a parent who was a smoker.
- Incidence of house dust mite allergy was much lower than expected.

Chemical fragrance

In the last three decades, there has been a massive explosion in the number of household products designed to fragrance your life. It started in the 1950s, when fabric conditioners were invented. Initially, they were designed to prevent static, but after a while more and more fragrances were added. Now, we have plug-in air fresheners that pulse fragrance into our rooms, air fresheners in our cars, fragrances that come out as we vacuum. We have polishes, cleaning sprays, fragranced bleaches, incense sticks, fragranced diffusers and fragranced candles, just to name a few of the culprits. Many people now spray something to make their room smell fresh rather than open a window. The fact that most homes are now double glazed means all these chemicals are sealed in and cannot drift away.

It is relatively simple to rid your home of chemical fragrances and it is essential if you and your child have chest and nasal symptoms. Fairly expensive perfume is not usually a problem. While cheap body sprays [e.g. Impulse, Charlie], inexpensive perfume [e.g. Next, Marks and Spencer] and after-shaves [e.g. Lynx] usually cause problems.

If you like the expensive perfume you wear, it is probably alright for you. But, if you share an office with someone whose perfume makes you feel sick or gives you a headache, this may be part of your chest or nasal problems.

Cigarette smoke

If your child suffers from asthma, catarrh or rhinitis, the chances are your smoking habit is aggravating their condition. It is not as simple a solution as ensuring you do not smoke in their presence, though that would undoubtedly help. The smell of the smoke will linger in your hair and clothes. If you possibly can, stop smoking.

Feathers

If you or your child are allergic to feathers, and feathers are present in pillows or duvets, symptoms are likely to be worse at night or first thing in the morning. If you have a feather settee or coat, symptoms are going to be worse when sitting on the settee or wearing the coat. Change your duvets and pillows for hypoallergenic hollow fibre products. Consider replacing the settee or coat.

Perceived wisdom

Most people with asthma, catarrh and rhinitis will presume, or have been told, there is little they can do to improve their condition, apart from regularly using inhalers and nasal sprays, because the main causes are pollution and house dust mite. But look where diesel, petrol and house dust mite, are on the list. Maybe it is not the pollution of the late 20th early 21st century that has led to asthma increase, but the fragrances we use to freshen our living spaces?

My recommendations are to:

- stop using fabric conditioners, plug-in air fresheners, fragranced bleach, polishes and cleaning sprays with additional fragrance, cheap perfumes, after-shaves and body butters. Looking at the figures I have presented above, these are the most important actions for you to take;
- remove feathers from your bedding and change feather cushions;
- stop smoking;
- sort out damp areas where you can;
- ensure good ventilation, open windows and consider cavity wall insulation to reduce effects of condensation and mould;
- seek expert damp advice; and
- clean obvious black mould with diluted bleach.

If you suspect pollens aggravate your condition, take note which time of the year your symptoms are worse. You may be allergic to any pollen, try when possible, to reduce your exposure. Never dry washing outside if your asthma, rhinitis, catarrh is worse in the summer. If you have spent a day outside and are struggling with rhinitis, catarrh or asthma, change your clothes, shower and wash your hair to reduce exposure. For more information about chemical fragrance, read *Chapter 16: Appendix*.

It can be a major problem for you, if you are allergic to your pet. If you can lower the load on other allergens or intolerances, such as food, fragrance, feathers, mould and cigarette smoke, this can sometimes enable you to cope better with your pet allergy.

Case Study

I was asked to see Adam when he was 14 months old. He had a constant green snotty nose, and there were some concerns around the possibility that he had a learning disability. As part of the investigations into this, he had been found to be quite significantly hard of hearing.

He had glue ear, which is when the build up of catarrh blocks the eardrum. He was due to have grommets inserted into both ears as soon as there was a suitable space at the local paediatric hospital.

On testing, I found Adam was intolerant of:

- cow's milk products;
- chemical fragrance; and
- mould.

He was still having two Cow and Gate [cow's milk based] feeds daily, and had been totally bottle fed since the age or four weeks.

Why these foods?	Cause
Cow's milk products	Frequency of use
Mould	Very damp flat

Adam's mother was happy to change Adam's milk feeds to a calcium supplemented alternative milk. Although these milks [e.g. rice, soya, coconut, almond, hazelnut, hemp or oat milks] are not considered suitable to provide a toddler with enough nutrition, Adam's mum was happy to change to one of these milks, because he was a very healthy eater, willing to try anything. I suggested Adam be given a daily children's multivitamin and mineral, and to ensure that any milk she chose for him was supplemented with calcium.

There was a major problem with damp in their newly bought flat, and it was getting worse. They had been considering getting the walls cavity insulated, and the results of testing kick started them into getting this job done. Meanwhile, I suggested that any black mould be removed using a dilute bleach. The tumble dryer in the flat did not have a proper extractor to outside. I encouraged her to remedy this, because that would be a major cause of the mould.

I advised his mum to start using fragrance free products in the home. She changed all her sprays, gave away the fragranced diffusers which she was using to counteract the damp smell, and stopped using Febreze.

Within two weeks Adam was free of catarrh, and could hear well. He did not need grommets inserting, and once he could hear well he seemed to 'wake up and take notice'. He passed all milestones at his next developmental check-up.

To recap
- Food intolerance is always linked to asthma, catarrh, cough and throat clearing.

- Reaction to fragrance in products, feathers and mould is much more common than reaction to house dust mite, petrol or diesel fumes.

Chapter 8: Fatigue, anxiety and depression

You may be surprised to hear the above symptoms can be caused by a reaction to food. But they sometimes are! There are many possible causes though, and a person's depression or anxiety might be due to a combination of all of them, including food intolerance.

- Life events which cause major stress, can lead to depression and anxiety. Temporary usage of anti-depressants and anti-anxiety medicines can help in the short term.
- A low level of Serotonin can lead to depression. SSRI anti – depressants can really help. Psychotherapy, cognitive behavioural therapy or counselling can be very effective.
- Irritability and mood swings are worse when someone is tired or unwell and most adults who are food intolerant feel tired and lethargic.
- Certain nutritional deficiencies can pre-dispose to depression and anxiety.
- Certain nutritional deficiencies can lead to pre-menstrual syndrome.
- Food intolerance can be a cause of depression, anxiety and pre-menstrual syndrome.

Read *Chapter 15; Recommended diet for your age and gender* in case food intolerance is part of the picture for you.

Case Study

Donna had been depressed for most of her adult life. She had been on and off anti-depressants for 20 years, since a termination of pregnancy when she was 21. She came to me for testing and advice about her IBS, and was surprised to learn from me that some cases of depression can be related to a food intolerance.

On testing, I found Donna was intolerant of:

- yeast;
- all cheeses;
- all yogurts; and
- tea.

And she was deficient in:

- vitamin B6.

Donna drank five teas most days, ate bread twice daily and frequently ate yogurt or fromage frais twice daily.

Why those foods?	Cause
Yeast	Frequency of use
Tea	Frequency of use
Why then?	**Trigger**
Termination of pregnancy	Hormonal and stress

Donna's IBS symptoms abated in just under a week. She started taking a vitamin B6 supplement. She then decided she would like to assess if she could cope without anti-depressants. I advised that she must cut back on dosage and frequency of her anti-depressant over a month or two, which Donna did following advice from her GP. From then, it seemed Donna could manage her depression with a dietary change and a vitamin B6 supplement. She did admit her many sessions of cognitive behavioural therapy over the years, and the strategies she had learned there had undoubtedly aided her recovery.

Vitamin B6 deficiency

If you suffer from PMS, depression or anxiety you are probably deficient in vitamin B6. For more information read *Chapter 16: Appendix*.

Panic attacks

If you experience panic attacks, read *Chapter 16: Appendix*. A vitamin B6 supplement can help.

Pre-menstrual syndrome

If you suffer PMS, take Evening Primrose Oil 1000mg daily.

Fatigue and lethargy

A huge majority of my adult clients are tired and many are lethargic. It is a common side effect of eating foods to which they are intolerant. Making appropriate dietary changes leads to considerable reduction in fatigue and lethargy. If my recommended change of diet does not help these symptoms, please go to your family doctor, if you have not already done so. Blood tests to check for anaemia and thyroid function might be necessary.

There are certain people who have a more severe problem, and these people find they are still tired despite a change of diet and having been checked for anaemia and a low functioning thyroid gland.

If you are; tired a lot of the time, have had a period of prolonged stress, crave salty foods, and surprisingly experience a second wind in the late evening; take a look at this website www.adrenalfatigue.org or read *Adrenal Fatigue, The 21st Century Stress Syndrome* by Dr James Wilson. There are good questionnaires, information about tests, and advice about how to deal with this condition. These symptoms occur when you are overstressed, causing you to use too much adrenaline, and as a consequence reduces your cortisol levels.

It is possible to get saliva tests to measure cortisol. In the UK these are not provided by the NHS. You will need to modify the way you eat, reduce your stress levels and take some supplements. Specialist advice from a qualified nutritionist is the best way to go, because they can organize the required tests for you. Make sure the nutritionist is BANT, British Association of Nutritional Therapy, registered, or equivalent [www.bant.org.uk].

Case Study

Vicky had suffered from Chronic Fatigue Syndrome for many years before I tested her. She seemed to be in remission, in that she had been bed bound at one stage, and was back at work part-time. But she was exhausted all the time. Vicky was lethargic, and had not found her 'get up and go.'

On testing, I found Vicky was intolerant of:

- coffee; and
- cocoa.

Why those foods?	Cause
Coffee	Frequency of use
Cocoa	Close relative of coffee
Why then?	Trigger
Starting the pill	Hormonal

Vicky used coffee to try to wake herself up, and to give her more energy. She regularly consumed eight strong mugs daily. She did not eat chocolate often. I explained that when coffee is a severe intolerance, cocoa [being a very close relative of coffee] can give similar symptoms. Vicky was very uneasy about stopping coffee, as it had proved to be such a prop for her flagging energy levels. I explained that every time the level of coffee in her blood dropped, she would crave some more, and when she had her 'fix' would feel better ... for a while ... until she needed her next 'fix'.

Vicky wondered whether it would be possible to still drink coffee if it was decaffeinated. I explained about the incidence of people I test who have a problem with decaff...95%. I advised her not to use decaffeinated products and just to stop the coffee.

We agreed Vicky's best way forward would be to cut down by one or two mugs of coffee daily until she was coffee free. This she managed, but not without difficulty. She definitely felt worse before she started feeling better. She had severe head and muscle aches, especially towards the end of the first week.

Ten days after she started reducing her coffee intake, Vicky was much more energetic, and enjoying her life again.

To recap

- Fatigue and lethargy are extremely common symptoms of food intolerance in adults.
- Depression and anxiety can be exacerbated or caused by food intolerance.
- Certain vitamin and mineral deficiencies are part of the picture for people who suffer depression, anxiety and pre-menstrual syndrome.

Chapter 9: Child behaviour problems

Might your 'difficult' child be food intolerant?

A sk yourself these questions.

1. Does your child suffer from any of the common physical symptoms of food intolerance? E.g. eczema, rashes, itch, headaches, tummy aches, loose stools, constipation. asthma, catarrh, rhinitis and growing pains.
2. Does your child have dark circles below their eyes?

Answered yes to both? If so, then I would try a change of diet. Read on for the most likely suspects.

What are the symptoms to look out for?

Below are the common manifestations of behaviour problems that can improve with a food intolerance approach.

Hostile, cannot be pleased, temper tantrums, irritable, moody
Easily upset, inattentive, disruptive
Short attention span, difficulty in concentration, poor school performance, difficulty in reading
Bullying, fighting, hurting people
Over-talkative, explosive speech, constantly interrupting, 'silly' or 'baby' talk
Argumentative, oppositional
Cannot keep still, restless, finger tapping, clothes irritate [e.g. waistbands]
Clumsiness, lack of coordination
Tired, weak, listless, depressed, tearful, anxious

Case Study

Chloe, aged 10, was brought to see me by her mother to see if I could find out the cause of her tummy aches. They were happening two or three times a week, and sometimes necessitated her leaving lessons. On questioning her, Chloe was extremely chatty and confident, inclined to interrupt in a way that became irritating after a while. She was articulate about her tummy pains, giving vivid description of their severity. Her mum said that she was a real 'drama queen', and it was sometimes difficult to know whether Chloe was exaggerating the pain.

When I asked how things were at school, both mother and daughter did disclose that Chloe had trouble making and maintaining friendships. I did not want to discuss this in detail in front of Chloe, so I had a telephone conversation with her mum that evening. From this conversation I elicited that Chloe was always in trouble in the classroom...calling out, interrupting, showing off, and complaining that other children were annoying her. At home, this middle child of three was 'ruling the roost,' getting her own way by virtue of her strong personality.

On testing, Chloe's food intolerances were:

- apple; and
- cocoa.

She had been eating two apples a day, and also drank copious amounts of apple juice. Chloe loved chocolate, and was allowed Nutella chocolate spread and a hot chocolate every day.

Why those foods?	Cause
Apple	Frequency of use
Cocoa	Frequency of use

Within two days Chloe's tummy aches were no longer an issue, all gone! But the added bonus was she was so much calmer. Gone were the constant interruptions, silly talk and loud behaviour. Her drama queen tendencies were still there, but her mum reported her teacher had really noticed a difference, in that Chloe was no longer craving the spotlight all the time. It took a while for friendships to build up, but her mum said Chloe was more able to take advice and listen to suggestions from her parents and friends. Family life was much less acrimonious.

If your child has been diagnosed with Attention Deficit Disorder, Attention Deficit Hyperactivity Disorder, you consider that he or she is 'hyper' some or all of the time, or you are struggling against the odds to get your child to behave, a change of diet can be helpful.

According to my 2012 Study, there was a 88% average improvement.

It is the perceived wisdom among parents, grandparents and teachers, that it is the additives and E numbers in junk food that are the major cause of problems in child behaviour. And yes, most people have a tale to tell of the child who changes from being amenable to 'climbing the walls' when given coca cola, other fizzy drinks or sweets. Many people blame sugar, [sugar rush] for their child's poor behaviour at a party.

But take a look at this...the results from my 2015 Survey of 18 children with behaviour problems.

Food	Percentage
Cow's milk	100
Sweet artificial flavours	60
Orange	50
Cocoa	45
Aspartame	40
E150 dark brown food colour	30

Points to note

- The 'worst' food was milk.
- Coming in a close second were sweet artificial flavours.
- Artificial colours showed up in only 30% of children, and then it was the dark brown colour, caramel, not the bright reds, yellows and greens.
- I have only tested one child in 21 years who was intolerant of sugar, and she did not have behaviour problems.

I therefore ask whether it is not 'sugar rush' or artificial colours that cause behaviour and concentration problems in children, but cow's milk products and the artificial flavours, which are commonly in sweet and coloured products.

Cow's milk, cheese and yogurt are all considered healthy foods, yet it is these foods that are the most common causes of behaviour problems. Most of the common fruit yogurts and drinks have far less fruit than they used to. Artificial fruit flavours have been added to these products.

Sweet artificial flavours

The use of sweet artificial flavours has exploded in the last five or so years, as a:

- method of improving flavour in cheap products;
- way to increase profit margins by using less or no fruit in a yogurt, sweet or drink; and
- way to keep prices low.

Is 'bad' behaviour always down to food?

Trying to help children who display these kind of behaviours is difficult, but it is even more important than it is with 'normal' children, to ensure you are consistent in what you expect, and the boundaries of what is allowable are clear to your child. Yes, I know it is not easy, especially with a child who is stroppy, moody, antagonistic and argumentative.

There is an excellent series of books about managing your child's behaviour written by the paediatrician, Dr Christopher Green: *Toddler Taming, Beyond Toddlerdom,* and *The Pocket Guide to Understanding ADHD.* These books are well worth a look. They are very sensible and down to earth.

What about your child?

There can be a massive range in differences in behaviour exhibited by children who are reacting adversely to something they are eating or drinking. These range from the 'severe' end of the spectrum, diagnosed Attention Deficit Disorder, Attention Deficit Hyperactivity Disorder, Oppositional Defiance Disorder, Pathological Demand Avoidance Syndrome, and their close relatives. The nomenclature of these diagnoses are always changing. Or your child may be stroppy, argumentative, rude, defiant, unable to keep still, and struggling to concentrate.

Such children tend to generate attention to themselves, at home or in the classroom, and often the 'normal' interventions in regard to expectations of good behaviour, ignoring 'bad' behaviours, and rewarding the child when he is 'good', do not work easily.

Other interventions

I have found the majority of children whom I test with behaviour problems have specific vitamin and mineral deficiencies. Taking supplements of these is a big part of the process of improvement for the child. Use these supplements if you see some, but not massive improvement following a change of diet.

Vitamin B6 supplementation
- Child aged 4 – 6   15mg
- Child aged 7 – 10   20mg
- Child aged 11 – 15   30 - 60mg, depending on age and size
- 16 years +   80mg

Vitamin B6 tablet dosage start at 40mg. Ensure that tablets are milk free. Lower doses come in drop form from www.biocare.co.uk.

Zinc supplementation
- 1 - 3 years   5mg/day
- 4 - 8 years   7mg/day
- 9 - 13 years   10mg/day
- 14 - 18 years   15mg/day

Zinc tablet dosage is normally in 15mg tablets. Ensure tablets are milk free. Lower dosages come in drop form from www.biocare.co.uk.

Essential fatty acids supplementation
Equazen Eye Q. For first 12 weeks three teaspoons of liquid per day with food. Thereafter one teaspoon daily. The flavouring of the liquid is natural lemon. Or Equazen Eye Q capsules six per day for the first 12 weeks, and then two per day thereafter.

Chromium supplementation
If your child's behaviour or concentration seems worse when he/she is hungry or has done a lot of exercise, he/she may be deficient in the mineral chromium. This mineral is responsible for keeping a person's blood sugar level stable.

If this is the case with your child he/she would benefit from eating more frequently, having a snack before indulging in after school sport, and eating foods that help to keep his/her blood sugar at a moderate level. Dips in blood sugar can lead such children to have meltdowns. Many of these children are sugar-obsessed. Eating sugary products does not keep blood sugar up for long, so eating sweet things often mean that the child is boomeranging between having a high blood sugar, and one that has dropped down too low, with resulting symptoms of irritability, mood swings, sometimes nausea, all of which go away when he/she eats.

To find out more about foods that keep blood sugar stable research the Glycaemic Index and the Glycaemic Load diet. In more severe cases a supplement of chromium may be necessary.

Case Study

George was a sullen looking nine year old. He argued the toss about everything. He was struggling in the school playground because of his temper, and consequently found it very hard to make friends. 'They just try to wind me up mum.' In the classroom he was not reaching his true potential because of his inability to concentrate. In a telephone call before bringing him for testing his mother said that she was at her wits end, because none of the strategies to encourage good behaviour that had worked well with her other children proved any use at all with George. Ritalin medication was being considered for George, and his mum brought him to be tested as a last ditch act of desperation before starting the medication.

George was minimally moving all the time that I was testing him... drumming his fingers, swinging on the chair, saying that his school trousers were uncomfortable round his middle, and wriggling his torso to try to get more comfortable. His speech came in bursts, like mini explosions, and despite being constantly reminded, George kept on interrupting while his mother was talking. When answering my questions George used a 'baby' voice, suitable for someone much younger than his years.

On testing, I found George reacted to:

- cow's milk products;
- aspartame;
- blackcurrant; and
- sweet artificial flavours.

George loved milk, cheese and yogurt. These foods had been actively encouraged, as he was a really 'picky' eater'. Aspartame was in every sugar free squash George had...five or more daily. Blackcurrant was his favourite flavour. Sweet artificial flavours were in every yogurt that he ate [three a day] his blackcurrant squash [up to three a day], and in the lemonade or coca cola that he was allowed as a treat at the weekends.

Why those foods?	Cause
Cow's milk products	Frequency of use
Sweet artificial flavours	Frequency of use
Blackcurrant	Frequency of use
Aspartame	Frequency of use

It proved impossible to discuss with George a change of diet, as he became a ball of anger, shouting and screaming. So his mum and I had a telephone conversation that evening. George was extremely angry about his change of diet, but his parents held firm, and within 48 hours he was a different boy. His parents estimate of the improvement at both home and school was 85%. Once he had been on supplements of vitamin B6, zinc and EyeQ essential fatty acid supplement, things improved still further. He could concentrate, he stopped fiddling. He never needed the Ritalin.

He did manage to reintroduce all foods apart from the sweet artificial flavours after three months exclusion, without any behavioural disturbance. They followed my advice to keep using alternative milks and squashes, and he did not redevelop any new intolerances, but every time the supplements were stopped, within less than a week George's behaviour went downhill.

If your child gets some, but not wonderful improvement with a change of diet, it may be worth considering if he has a condition called pyroluria.

Pyroluria

Pyroluria is a disorder which is often familial, and occurs with stress. It is a biochemical imbalance in which kryptopyroles [a by product of haemoglobin synthesis] are produced. These are excreted in the urine, but unfortunately have the action that they bind with vitamin B6 and zinc. Therefore, available vitamin B6 and zinc is passed out in the urine, and deficiencies result. In children this manifests itself as problems with behaviour, mood, irritability, poor stress control and poor anger control.

It is possible to confirm your child is pyroluric by doing a urine test. This can be ordered by a nutritional therapist. Make sure that the person you choose is registered. In the UK this will mean BANT registered [The British Association of Nutritional Therapists] or a nutritionally qualified doctor.

Follow this link for doctors who have training/experience in naturopathy or nutritional therapy in the UK. http://www.biolab.co.uk/index.php/cmsid__biolab_medical_referral_list

Treatment of pyroluria is by supplementing vitamin B6 and zinc. If the symptoms are mild to moderate, symptoms will improve within a week or two. If severe, then symptoms can take a few months to improve. If the supplementation is discontinued, symptoms will usually return within a few weeks. It will be necessary to continue indefinitely.

To recap
- If your child has dark under eye shadows, he is likely to be food intolerant.
- If your child has other symptoms of food intolerance, then food could also be affecting his behaviour.
- Cow's milk products are nearly always implicated in child behaviour problems.
- Sugar is rarely a cause, but sweet artificial flavours commonly are.
- Severe cases will benefit from supplementing zinc, vitamin B6 and essential fatty acids.

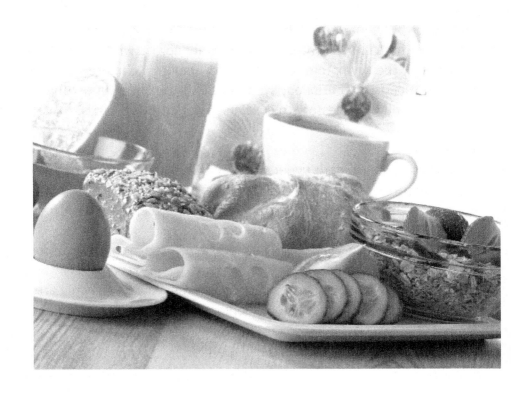

Part 3: Common Misconceptions

Chapter 10: Milk or lactose?

Confusion reigns with many people about the definition of lactose. Many think that milk and lactose are synonymous. They are not. Take a look at these case histories which illustrate this well.

Case Study

Ten year old Josie was having a horrible time with her stomach. When she was eight she had started having regular daily pains. These were pretty severe and meant she could not concentrate in the classroom and often needed to go home. After nine months of suffering, Josie had an endoscopy, which is a procedure where a camera was placed into her stomach while she was under sedation. Following the endoscopy, her parents were told she was lactose intolerant. They were advised to only give Josie lacto free products.

Josie improved to a certain extent. The severe stomach pains only occurred once a fortnight, but day in, day out, she felt uncomfortable. However, she was missing very little school and the family settled down to the fact her stomach was better than it had been before her new diet.

In 2013, I tested her dad and he was very pleased with the results and on the back of this I was asked to see Josie.

On testing, I found Josie was intolerant of:

- cow's milk products.

I recommended Josie stop using the Lactofree products for ten days and see how her stomach reacted to this change, before trying one day of using the Lactofree milk products again. During this time, she was to use other alternatives to cow's milk. I advised she not be given goat's nor sheeps' products because they contain lactose. Within two days

Josie's stomach discomfort was gone. But ten days later it returned on the day she tried Lactofree milk. Josie therefore, followed a cow's milk free diet for three months. After which she tolerated the reintroduction of cow's milk, cheese and yogurt and has remained fine on restricted frequency and amounts only twice a day. She has continued to use coconut milk and almond milk for cereals and milk shakes.

Are lactose intolerance and cow's milk intolerance the same thing?

No they are not despite what most people think. Lactose is milk sugar which is just one part of cow's milk.

Most of my milk intolerant clients have heard of Lactofree products. A high percentage of them presume Lactofree products will be a suitable alternative for cow's milk. Most of them will have someone encouraging them to use Lactofree because and I quote, 'It tastes just like milk.'

If someone is truly lactose intolerant, it is because they do not have enough lactase enzyme produced by their small intestine. This means they cannot digest lactose. It will cause them pain, nausea and quite often diarrhoea as well. Lactofree milk is normal milk, hence the normal taste, but it has the enzyme lactase added. If a patient is definitely lacking lactase, symptoms will improve, because the enzyme will enable adequate digestion of lactose. However, if the person is intolerant of cow's milk, using Lactofree will not rid them of symptoms completely.

Josie was given a diagnosis of lactose intolerance and her symptoms did improve, but she was also reacting to other parts of cow's milk. It was not until she avoided all cow's milk products that she felt better.

This next case study is slightly different, but it is a common story.

Case Study

Alice, also aged ten, came to see me because she had been suffering stomach aches, nausea and diarrhoea for 18 months. After several visits to her GP she was referred to a paediatrician. Meanwhile Alice was missing school far too often and was becoming increasingly anxious about her stomach.

The paediatrician suggested on the basis of the history, that Alice was lactose intolerant. He suggested Alice be fed on Lactofree milk, cheeses, yogurts and margarines and return six weeks later. He explained, the sugars in milk, the lactose, are the worst part of milk and the other bits of milk, including proteins, and fat, are rarely a problem.

There was very little improvement for Alice and because of her overt anxiety, the doctor felt it was time for her to see a child psychiatrist.

The following week I met Alice. Yes, she was an anxious ten year old and she was feeling extremely unwell, constantly nauseous, with urgent diarrhoea, which worried her at school. Also she was concerned about the prospect of transferring to high school three months later, when she felt so unwell.

On testing, I discovered Alice was intolerant of:

- cow's milk products.

I recommended she stop using Lactofree items and change to the other alternatives I suggested. Within 36 hours Alice felt better. There was no need for child psychiatry. All her anxiety was gone.

To recap
- Lactose intolerance and cow's milk intolerance are not the same thing.

- Even if someone has been diagnosed as lactose intolerant, either by blood test, endoscopy or hydrogen breath test, when their symptoms have not gone completely, it is worth trying complete cow's milk avoidance to see if symptoms improve.

Chapter 11: Wheat intolerance. Myth, fact or yeast?

Wheat and gluten intolerance is, according to nearly every website, newspaper and magazine, massively increasing in the western world. To provide gluten free and wheat free food for all these people is big business.

Why are less than 1% of my clients intolerant of wheat, and less than 0.25% of gluten?

Many people have a big suspicion of wheat as part of their health problem, and some of those will already have tried a wheat free diet before they see me for testing. Mostly they will have seen some improvement in their symptoms, but the majority will say they know that it is not the full picture for them.

Many people who come to me for testing, and who think that they are wheat intolerant, suffer from Irritable Bowel Syndrome symptoms or indigestion. These days should one talk to a friend, read a newspaper article or magazine, go online for information, or talk to a family doctor, the global suggestion will be...try a wheat/gluten free diet, because the perception is wheat is a really common food intolerance.

When people are in the process of considering a wheat/gluten free diet to alleviate tummy symptoms, they will very often look at what they eat over a period of a week or so, and try to make a judgement of whether wheat might be a factor.

Let us take a look at a sufferer's typical day's food and drink, the symptoms suffered, and his subsequent conclusions.

Food and drink	Symptom	Conclusion
7.30am On waking	Loose stools x 3	Do not know
7.45am Tea		
8.00am Weetabix		
11.00am Coffee	Bloating started	Wheat in Weetabix
13.00pm Tea Cheese sandwich Satsuma Salt and vinegar crisps	Bloating increases	Wheat in Weetabix and in sandwich
14.00pm Coffee		
15.00pm Chocolate	Tummy ache	
17.00pm Tea	Bloating worse Loose stool Wind +++	Too much wheat
19.00pm Supper Salmon Potatoes Broccoli Yogurt Coffee	Very tired Awful bloating	Broccoli

This person was not intolerant of wheat, but of milk. There was milk in every hot drink that he had consumed, milk with the Weetabix, cheese in the cheese sandwich, milk in the chocolate and yogurt, and butter on all the vegetables.

If it was not for the fact everyone had sowed the seed of wheat being a common intolerance, he might not even have considered wheat could be part of the picture.

Looking at it from another angle, one where any frequent food can be the culprit, his problem foods and drinks could just as easily have been yeast [in bread and crisps] a preservative in bread, or tea or coffee [three of each daily].

Sometimes, when someone excludes wheat, they reduce or avoid other possible causes, as below.

- They stop eating bread to avoid wheat, and as a result avoid yeast and the common preservatives.
- They stop eating pizza, to avoid wheat, and therefore avoid yeast and cheese too.
- They stop eating pasta and may as a result consume less cheese.
- They stop having wheat based cereals and therefore use less milk.

If other foods apart from wheat are the problem, and they eat less of them by avoiding wheat, their symptoms are less and they think that wheat is their problem food. They tell their friends, or post it on an online forum, and the wheat myth continues.

The other thing to bear in mind with gut symptoms is that grains, vegetables, fizzy drinks, spices, pulses, onions and alcohol can all sometimes be a bit much for a troubled gut to cope with. People cut out these food groups, and are also often advised to do so by their doctors.

When the underlying food cause is found, the person can manage all these foods without adverse symptoms. And for those who still cannot digest these foods, taking digestive enzymes can be helpful.

Recently a friend of mine asked for my advice about his tummy symptoms. He lived too far away to get to me soon for a test. Mike thought that when he ate wheat, he would usually get a bad tummy ache within half an hour, and then would need to rush to the toilet, where his stool would be abnormally loose. But this did not happen every time.

Because I could not test him for a while I asked him if he would mind being a guinea pig for me. Initially I asked Mike to avoid yeast, all cheeses and all yogurts for a week. This allowed him to use wheat in wraps, soda bread, some crispbreads, scones and cake. His tummy aches happened every time he ate any of those things. Mike's assumption about wheat was therefore understandable.

But knowing that such a small percentage of people whom I test actually are wheat intolerant, I started wondering about additives.

I compared the ingredients that were in his preferred wheat and gluten free bread, the wraps, soda bread, and his previously preferred normal bread. They all contained an emulsifier E471 [mono and diglycerides of fatty acids]. E471 and its close relative E472 [a-f] is used as a preservative in many baked goods. The gluten free bread contained a different preservative E282 [Calcium Proprionate].

I suggested Mike try a wheat based bread that did not contain E471. He did, and suffered no symptoms. E471 is also in many margarines, so it would explain why Mike had similar symptoms when he ate bought cake. I suggested that he used butter or spreadable butter instead of margarine.

Case Study

I met Pamela when she was 71, when she had been suffering from bowel symptoms for 11 years. Like many people, Pam had tried changes to her diet to alleviate symptoms. She was suffering intermittent diarrhoea, loose stools and constipation. She was bloated most days, and got moderate to severe tummy pains at least three times a week.

Four years before I met Pam, a colonoscopy and blood tests had revealed nothing abnormal, and she had been given a diagnosis of Irritable Bowel Syndrome. Following hospital advice at the time she stopped drinking fizzy drinks and spicy food. She had been on a wheat and gluten free diet for two years. She avoided onions in any form. All vegetables gave her symptoms, so she rarely ate them. She was very suspicious of fruits, so did not eat much of that food group.

At one stage, before colonoscopy refuted the diagnosis, it had been suggested that she might have diverticulitis, so following some internet research, she had made sure that she never ate any pips or seeds [she would sieve tomatoes to remove the seeds].

She had started using lactofree foods, in case lactose intolerance was part of her problem.

To make things more complicated, Pam was a strict vegetarian. She did eat fish very occasionally but she really did not like eggs.

As a consequence of all these changes her diet was pretty bland, and not very healthy at all. Despite those massive changes to her diet, she had seen only minimal improvements symptomatically. At the beginning of the testing procedure, I explained to her that, because there were so many foods that she had not eaten for so long, I might have to do a second session of testing a few days later, when she had eaten all of her problem foods. She was very uneasy about this, as she really did not want to risk the bad symptoms that vegetables, for example, tended to provoke. I explained that it was very common for IBS sufferers to suffer symptoms from vegetables and fruit, and that, when the underlying food cause [e.g. milk, yeast, tea, coffe] was avoided, then the vegetables, fruit, fizzy drinks and spices would not affect their gut. I also explained that my 2011 Study found that peoples' perceptions of their problem foods were only 17% accurate.

Eventually we compromised, and she decided she would strictly avoid the foods that I suggested for a week to ten days. When she was asymptomatic, she would introduce the foods she had suspected were bad for her. If she wished, at that stage, I could test her a second time to confirm.

On initial testing, I found Pam was intolerant of:

- yeast;
- all cheeses;
- all yogurts; and
- hemp/linseeds.

The gluten free bread that she had been using contained yeast. Many of her specialist vegetarian products [e.g. quorn, smoked tofu] contained yeast, as did the breaded cod that she ate twice a week. In addition, the slimmer's vegetable soup that she used for lunch on many days of the week contained yeast as a savoury flavour.

She ate cheese daily. She ate yogurt twice daily. She put powdered hemp [linseeds] on cereal, and salads at least twice daily, to ensure she had more protein.

Why those foods?	Cause
Yeast, all cheeses, all yogurts	Frequency of use
Hemp/linseeds	Frequency of use
Why then?	Trigger
We never worked out what the trigger was	

These were the underlying cause of her symptoms, and the vegetables that she strongly suspected were actually 'red herrings'.

Pam and I tried to work out how, without cheese and the powdered hemp, she could have enough protein in her diet. She decided she would eat nuts, of as many varieties as she could find, and she would experiment with pulses when her tummy had settled.

Pamela's tummy symptoms were massively improved after a week on the exclusion diet, apart from the occasions on which she ate broccoli or cauliflower.

What foods might it be when someone suspects wheat?

When a person suspects wheat is an issue for them, it is usually because another food or additive has been eaten with wheat.

Let us consider what foods might be mixed with wheat in, e.g. bread, biscuits, cake, wraps, soda bread, and cereals.

Here are the percentages of people with IBS who reacted adversely to such foods in 2015.

Foods	Percentage
Yeast in bread croissants pizza	30
Cheese on pasta, in pizza, in a sandwich	30
E471/2, an emulsifier in many breads, margarine, cakes, wraps	7
E282, a preservative in many breads, wraps, cakes, soda bread	2
Soya, in most bread, bought cakes, vegetarian and vegan food	2
Raising agents in cake, wraps, soda bread, crispbreads, biscuits	1

Anyone suffering symptoms after eating these foods might think they were intolerant of wheat.

If you are reacting to an ingredient in bread it is 30 times more likely to be yeast than wheat.

More about yeast

A substantial number of people who I test react adversely to the food group comprising yeast, all cheeses and all yogurts. When yeast is a problem for you, all cheeses and all yogurts will also be involved. Only one person in 2015 had a yeast intolerance without also having reactions to cheese and yogurts.

In fact, 30% of the adults in my 2015 Survey reacted adversely to yeast, all cheese and all yogurt.

Yeast intolerance and candida

With the internet making access to information so easy, and blogs and anecdotal stories masquerading as valid advice, many people are led to believe that yeast intolerance and candida are one and the same thing. I often receive an email from a client who is yeast intolerant to say that they have looked it up on the internet and found that they need to be on a much stricter diet than I suggested.

Many people think that candidiasis is synonymous with a yeast intolerance, and I agree that the two conditions are connected.

In my experience, most people who are intolerant to baker's yeast do not have candidiasis. I am confident about that statement because 90% of my clients with a yeast intolerance recover from their original symptoms after one week on my suggested diet, without needing to follow the very difficult restrictions of an anti-candida diet. I have noted other useful signposts for candida problems. When on testing, I find a client is intolerant to yeast, all cheese and all yogurt plus all alcohol and sugar, they do not feel well on my suggested exclusion diet alone. These people account for 1% of those with a baker's yeast intolerance. They are candidiasis sufferers.

Candidiasis is not as common as the internet might suggest.

Who might be a candidiasis sufferer?

The people most likely to have a candida issue are those who have:
- gut symptoms, and any other symptoms of food intolerance;
- brain fog;
- recurrent thrush and/or athletes foot or any other fungal infections; and
- taken frequent courses of antibiotics, especially long term courses.

Antibiotics however, can be a trigger for food intolerances to begin. Do not automatically assume that having been prescribed antibiotics means you are suffering from candidiasis.

What is candidiasis?

Whole books have been written on this subject, one of the first and still the best of which is *The Yeast Connection* by William Crook.

Candidiasis is an overgrowth of the yeast [fungus] candida, usually because the good bacteria that habitually live in our guts have been killed off by antibiotics or possibly steroids. Once the good bacteria have been killed off, the candida fungus grows to take their place. This can lead to 'leaky gut' which means small molecules of food escape through the gut walls. This leads to adverse symptoms being suffered in other parts of the body. Be aware also, that a simple food intolerance can also lead to many and varied symptoms.

In my 2015 Survey, there was only one person who I suspected suffered from candidiasis. The proof of the pudding, for me, is that if someone is asymptomatic on a yeast free, all cheese free, all yogurts free diet, then they cannot be suffering from candidiasis. If they did have candidiasis they would not feel better on an exclusion diet alone.

Things can only improve for a candidiasis sufferer when he/she avoids:
- yeast, all cheeses, all yogurts;
- sugar;
- all alcohol; and
- mushrooms.

And reduces:
- fruit intake, especially fruit juices and dried fruit.

And takes:
- probiotics; and
- Medication that kills the candida fungus off completely.

My advice to anyone who I suspect has candidiasis is to consult a qualified nutritionist who in the UK are BANT [British Association of Nutritional Therapists] registered. This is really important to ensure that the sufferer is directed in detail to follow the correct diet, and to be advised on supplements which will enable a gut environment that discourages the growth of candida. A nutritionist can also advise on supplements that help to kill off the candida fungus.

To recap

- Yeast intolerance is 30 times more common than wheat intolerance.
- When the underlying food intolerance is correctly identified and avoided, the person can manage to eat the foods that they previously suspected.
- Yeast intolerance is not the same as candidiasis.

Chapter 12: Monosodium glutamate and sweet artificial flavouring

The monosodium glutamate story

Monosodium glutamate, known as MSG or E621, is the flavour enhancer found in many cheap restaurant and takeaway meals. The increase in its use in other foods, such as flavoured crisps and dehydrated products, including: pot noodles, cup-a-soups, packet casserole mixes and gravy granules, increased massively in the 1990s.

Gradually in the 2000s, MSG started to receive a bad name and many people, especially parents of young children, did not want to buy MSG products. In 2003, MSG affected one third of my clients. In 2011, the incidence dropped to 1 in 5 people. In 2015, the figure was only 9%.

The product introduced instead was a substance called hydrolysed vegetable protein. Any product containing this product was advertised as being 'additive-free', although my taste buds told me its taste was very similar to MSG. For a while, it was in many gravy powders, stock cubes, packet mixes e.g. chilli con carne, shepherd's pie, chicken chasseur and in one specific brand of stock powder, Marigold Swiss Vegetable Bouillon. Recently, the only product I can find it in, is the Marigold stock powder.

In 2011, 31% of my clients were intolerant of hydrolysed vegetable protein and in my last survey, less than 1%. These figures seem to directly correlate with a reduction in the number of products, which now contain HVP.

The other food increasingly used to flavour savoury edible products instead of MSG is yeast. It is in many gravies, stock cubes and gels and most flavoured crisps. This enables the manufacturers to claim 'no artificial flavourings'. Between 2002 and 2015, the incidence of yeast intolerance in adults has grown from 14% to 30%, which may stem from the increase in its use to replace MSG and HVP.

In the last few years many flavoured crisps, microwave noodles and microwaveable savoury rice dishes have started to include different chemicals which do the same job as MSG. They provide cheap savoury flavour. They all have E numbers that directly follow on from E621 or MSG. These numbers are E622–E635 inclusive. For more information read *Chapter 16: Appendix.*

These additives are used with increasing frequency in noodles, flavoured crisps, gravy, stock cubes and gels and are allowed to market themselves as 'free from monosodium glutamate.'

Case Study

I saw Arun because his eczema had flared up as his A levels got closer. He always had eczema, but it was usually only a little itchy in the creases of his knees and elbows. By the time he came to see me, it had spread to his face, chest, arms and legs and was driving him crazy. He was a well-built sporty lad, who liked to show off his physique in the summer and was looking forward to a post A level trip to Ibiza. However, his skin was so bad, he really did not want to go.

On testing, I found Arun was intolerant of:

• orange; and
• monosodium glutamate.

Arun loved orange juice and drank it daily. He knowingly had monosodium glutamate in a chinese takeaway meal about once a fortnight. I told him the sort of products that MSG was likely to be in and encouraged him and his mother to read labels on everything he ate, to exclude MSG.

Why these foods?	Cause
Orange	Frequency of use
Monosodium glutamate	Frequency of use
Why then?	**Trigger**
A Level examinations	Stress

I recommended measures to help him, including that his clothes be washed in Surcare, that no fabric conditioner be used, and that shower gels, shampoos and soaps be changed to the brand Simple.

I advised a zinc supplement to correct a zinc deficiency.

A week later, Arun was little improved, so I asked him to return for more testing. I asked him to bring with him anything that he ate regularly that contained multiple ingredients. At this stage I sometimes find that someone has, in error, been eating a problem food inadvertently, or I find a new problem food.

This was the case for Arun. We checked the cereals, cereal bars, ketchup, mayonnaise, biscuits, cake, sweets, fizzy drinks and one brand of crisps he was eating and found they were all fine. I tested the microwave noodles he had as a snack every afternoon when he walked in from school. This product contained E627 or disodium guanylate. I advised him to avoid all additives with E numbers between E622 and E635, because they perform a similar function to monosodium glutamate or E621.

Later Arun found another brand of crisps he was eating contained E622 or monopotassium L glutamate. Four days after excluding these his eczema was nearly gone, he had no new patches and no itch. Two weeks after that his skin was normal, with a little bit of change in texture where the eczema had been at its worst.

From that time onwards, I routinely advise those who react adversely to MSG to also avoid E numbers E622–E635.

Case Study

Ezinne, a 64 year old Afro Caribbean lady, came for a test because she had stomach problems.

Daily bloating was so bad her size changed and she looked six months pregnant. She suffered loose stools and griping pains, preceding an urgent trip to the bathroom. She had numerous joint and muscle pains. The combination of these two sets of symptoms were affecting her quality of life severely, and she was unable to volunteer at her local church. This had been the centre of her working and social life. She was becoming depressed, said she felt old before her time. Ezinne did not have a healthy diet. She had a very sweet tooth and was borderline type two diabetic. She loved cake and ate it frequently as a meal replacement.

On testing, I discovered Ezinne was intolerant of:

- palm oil; and
- monosodium glutamate.

In line with her West Indian heritage, Ezinne used palm oil in cooking. It was in every cake she ate too. She tended to go for the cheap ranges, which commonly use palm oil. Many Afro Caribbeans use a stock cube called Maggi. Ezinne was no exception. For her regular meals a Maggi stock cube was used in a sauce and crumbled over the vegetables. Maggi contains monosodium glutamate and palm oil.

Why these foods?	Cause
Palm oil	Frequency of use
Monosodium glutamate	Frequency of use
Why then?	**Trigger**
We could not work out a trigger	

Within ten days of the eliminating these two ingredients, Ezinne was feeling perky! Her stomach had settled down and her aches and pains were gone, apart from her left thumb. She was welcomed back to her church with open arms!

The sweet flavouring story

In 2003, the flavouring in coca cola and sometimes lemonade were the only sweet flavours I found were a problem for my clients, usually only for those people who were drinking these daily. In the last six or seven years though, the proliferation in use of sweet chemical flavours has exploded. Flavours which were used only in penny sweets and products like bubble gum are now present in many more products, presumably to keep prices down and profits up.

In any month during 2003, I counted on the fingers of one hand the people who were not able to tolerate these flavours. Now, they affect 12% of my clients and 62.5% of the 13–18 year olds I test.

These artificial flavours can be in anything sweet, including products most people consider healthy, such as yogurt, sugar free squashes, lite juice drinks and children's medicines. They are in many gluten and wheat free sweet products, including cake and biscuits. They are labelled simply as 'flavour' or 'flavouring' with no E number, no specific chemical name or E number whatever the flavour is. This means people who might try to avoid E numbers will still be consuming these flavours. Read *Chapter 16: Appendix* for more about 'flavours'.

Case Study

Phoebe came to see me because a friend of hers had lost a lot of weight on a diet I had suggested. Phoebe had recently had a painful break-up with a long term boyfriend and thought no other young man was going to ever fancy her again. I am always careful to explain in these circumstances that weight loss is not something I can promise. However, many people lose weight on the diet I suggest because they are cutting out foods they love and of which they were having too much.

Phoebe was overweight by a couple of stone. She was three to four dress sizes bigger than she wished to be. This weight gain had started in her teens when she had for several years eaten really unhealthily, buying sweets, crisps and fizzy drinks on her way home from school.

Now 25 years old, she had decided to take herself in hand. Initially she tried the 5:2 diet, which allowed only 500 calories for two days every week, but she was feeling sick, shaky, headachy and irritable on those days and had given up that diet. Recently, she had joined Weightwatchers and in only two weeks had lost six pounds in weight.

On questioning, Phoebe admitted she suffered headaches several times a week and they were bad enough to necessitate taking a painkiller.

She told me she used skimmed milk in every cup of tea and coffee, two each per day and sometimes more on weekdays. Phoebe loved cheddar cheese, but knew it was fattening and since joining Weightwatchers, had been having cottage cheese every lunchtime.

In the past, sweet artificial flavours had been in all the sweets and fizzy drinks that she used. Recently, these flavours were in the low fat yogurts suggested for her Weightwatchers diet, as well as in the calorie free diet coke and diet lemonade she used regularly as a mixer.

Phoebe loved chocolate, but had not eaten it daily for quite a while. There had been sweet flavours in her preferred brand of chocolate.

Why these foods?	Cause
Cow's milk products	Frequency of use
Sweet artificial flavours	Frequency of use
Cocoa	Recent frequency of use
Why then?	**Trigger**
Relationship break up	Stress

I found Phoebe was deficient in chromium, which I explained was an underlying factor behind her sweet tooth, her headaches and why she had felt so unwell on the 5:2 diet.

Although Phoebe had come to have a test to assist her weight loss, she had a few added bonuses. She started sleeping through the night, something that had been rare since her mid-teens, and she was no longer constipated. When taking a chromium supplement and following my recommendations for keeping her blood sugar more stable, she no longer craved sweet foods.

For more information on chromium deficiency read *Chapter 5: Headache and migraine* and *Chapter 16: Appendix*.

Case Study

Charley aged 16, came to see me with her mum because she was getting really bad headaches every day. With school exams looming, she was beginning to panic, because she felt unwell most of the time. She was exhausted. She found eating sweet things made her feel better and temporarily gave her more energy. Her mother felt Charley was sugar addicted and had been fighting a losing battle to persuade Charley to eat more healthily. Charley said she felt even worse if she gave up sweet foods and drinks.

On testing, I found Charley was intolerant of:

• sweet artificial flavours;

although there was no problem with sugar itself or glucose.

Charley had a yogurt for breakfast with some orange or blackcurrant squash, a fizzy drink at break time, pizza and a chocolate muffin for lunch alongside another fizzy drink and sweets on the way home from school. Also, she had another yogurt and more squash in the evening. All of these food and drinks contain sweet artificial flavours, apart from the pizza.

Why these foods?	Cause
Sweet artificial flavours	Frequency of use
Why then?	Trigger
We could not work out a trigger	

I advised Charley she was likely to have worse symptoms than usual, including headaches and fatigue during the first few days on my recommended exclusion diet. I explained it was best for her to cut down on the sweet flavourings, to avoid feeling too ill, but she said she would rather stop eating and drinking them altogether and suffer the consequences, which she did!

Poor Charley felt very unwell, as though she had flu symptoms. She had to go to bed with the worst headache ever. She was extremely fatigued, lethargic and her muscles ached abominably.

Luckily though, only five days later Charley felt great! Her head was clear and she had her energy back. She was able to eat sweet things, including sweets, yogurts, cake, fizzy drinks and squashes, as long as she chose brands with no artificial flavours. The whole experience had scared her though and she decided to eat in a more healthy way in the future, with less sugar in her diet and more fruit and vegetables. Her mother was happy!

Sugar intolerance. Myth or fact?
According to my data a tiny percentage of people react to sugar itself even when the person eats sugar excessively [less than 1% of people tested in 2015]. When someone has a sweet tooth and uses sugar frequently the problem food or additive is usually something eaten with the sugar. This will be either sweet artificial flavours, as these are in most sweets, fizzy drinks, bought cakes, some squash, yogurts and chocolate, or dairy products such as in chocolate, ice cream, cake, toffees, fudge and custard.

To recap
- The food industry has invented new additives to take the place of monosodium glutamate.
- The use of sweet artificial flavours is increasing.
- Sugar is a rare intolerance even if eaten frequently.

Chapter 13: Alcohol

I rarely find anyone who has a problem with all alcohol. In my 2015 Survey there was only one person out of 345 adults, who reacted adversely to every form of alcohol. This one person had all the symptoms of an overgrowth of a fungus called candida, a condition called candidiasis. Read *Chapter 11: Wheat intolerance. Myth fact or yeast?*

However, many people develop a problem with their favourite wine, bitter, lager, spirit or mixer simply because of frequently drinking their favourite tipple! Sometimes a certain sort of wine, even if not often used, can be a problem. It can happen that someone who shares a bottle of wine without enthusiasm with a partner, because it is the partner's favourite, may be better off with a wine they actually enjoy.

But booze is complicated. It is a gastric irritant. Many people have suspicions of alcohol because it affects their gut adversely. Think about how a hangover can make you feel sick! However, sometimes, this can just be a red herring.

This chapter aims to illustrate how people are often wrong in their assumptions about alcohol by sharing with you ten case histories that reveal a different story.

Case Studies

> Paul was sure something around alcohol was a problem for him because he felt unaccountably hung over after even one drink. After coming to see me for food intolerance testing, it turned out to be the monosodium glutamate in the dry roasted peanuts he ate when he had a drink that was a problem for him. He ate these at home when friends came round for a meal, and when he had a beer in a bar after work.

Melissa's favourite drink was Pinot Grigio wine. She truly believed all alcohol gave her a headache. Luckily for her she was unaffected by any other alcoholic drink apart from Pinot Grigio.

Alan no longer suffers from gout since he stopped drinking port.

John loved drinking bitter. Every evening on his way home from work, he had a couple of pints of Young's beer. He kept this same routine for 20 years. His wife was convinced beer was at the root of all his health problems, but he did not want to know! In fact, he put off being tested because he did not want to find out that he was unable to drink beer any more. Amongst other symptoms, he was struggling to get a good night's sleep and his stomach felt very unsettled, windy and bloated. I tested him for many different bitters and lagers and found the only one that was a problem for him was Youngs! Poor John. From then on, he rung the changes with his beer, sometimes drinking John Smiths or Guinness or going for lager or gin. He sleeps soundly now and his stomach is much more settled, the bloating has completely gone, and it was not a beer belly after all!

Every time Simon had any kind of an alcoholic drink, his stomach felt appalling the next day. His indigestion was worse than normal, his stools were loose and sometimes the need to go to the bathroom was so urgent, he nearly had an accident. When he stopped eating cow's milk products and cocoa, his digestion settled and he coped with alcohol again. The underlying cause was cow's milk and the alcohol was the red herring.

Kelly just cannot drink red wine any more. She loves it, but every time she drinks it, she gets a flushed face, embarrassingly so and sneezes uncontrollably. Her partner still drinks red wine and is very picky about his choices. He loves Rioja and other heavy reds. Luckily for Kelly though, I discovered the lighter reds like Beaujolais and Pinot Noir suited her better and now, that is what she drinks! No sneezing and no red face any more.

Brad came to see me because he had developed arthritis at the age of 45. To start with, excluding heavy red wines helped him but he developed a problem with all red wines. I suggested he rotate the drinks he uses because he likes to drink alcohol three or four times a week. Now he sometimes has white wine or rose and he has found a taste for lager and vodka. He has realised that variety is the spice of life!

Janet found it hard to believe it was the flavouring in the tonic and not the gin that was causing her rashes.

Monique cannot stand Pinot Grigio wine and only drank Chardonnay if someone paid her! They both showed up in her testing and she will probably never be tempted to drink them again.

Darren's wife said she hated it when he came home after a Friday nights drink with the lads because he was so aggressive. His tipple was Stella. At my suggestion, drinking a different lager has made Darren a nicer person to know on a Friday night!

Chapter 14: Supposedly healthy 'clean' eating

Many people who come to me for a consultation are keen to tell me how healthily they eat. They eat fresh home cooked food, no ready meals, rarely eat red meat, reduced sugar and no fruit juice because of the sugar content. Not just five a day, but eight a day! No caffeine, few additives, etcetera.

My heart sinks at these conversations, because it is usually a hard sell to persuade them if they are intolerant to their healthy foods. Healthy eaters are just as likely to become intolerant to favourite and frequent foods. According to my figures, the most common food intolerances are dairy products, yeast and fruit, healthy foods really?

Additives

Additives are not the most common food intolerances, but many people are sure they are a cause of their symptoms. They try to eat an additive free diet and comb product labels and ingredient lists for E numbers. It is always surprising to people when it is not the additives that are the problem. Only 30% of adults are intolerant to the combined total of all the additives labelled with E numbers, which is lower than the percentage of people who suffer from a cow's milk intolerance, 35%.

The additive affecting the highest percentage of my clients is sweet artificial flavouring. This has no E number. Most people will not recognise it as an additive and therefore not attempt to avoid it, should they have strong opinions about additive avoidance. It is labelled as 'flavour' or 'flavouring', whatever the flavour it provides. The same word is used whether it tastes like a strawberry, cherry, orange, or lemon. It affects more than half the teenagers I test, because this age group homes in on products using artificial flavours, including fizzy drinks, sweets and alco-pops. However, these flavours are now in an increasing number of products considered to be healthy, e.g. yogurts, sugar free or no added sugar squashes and children's vitamins and medicines.

Sugar

Many people consider sugar the big baddie in our modern diets. Undoubtedly eating a lot of sweet foods is not great for healthy teeth, weight control or preventing Type 2 diabetes.

Sugar is rarely a food to which people become intolerant, despite the fact that it is a frequently used food for many of my clients. Less than 0.78% of people in my 2015 Survey were intolerant of sugar. This included people with a sweet tooth who were eating sugar in various forms many times in a day, making it a frequent food for them. I usually only test one person a year who is intolerant of sugar.

However, people with a sweet tooth who eat many sugar based foods might have a problem with dairy products or chocolate, as most of their sugar consumption is likely to be in products which are dairy rich, e.g. cake, ice cream, chocolate, toffee, fudge and custard. Or if sweets are their favoured way of consuming sugar, sweet artificial flavours might be the cause of their intolerance problems.

Many of these people are likely to be at risk of having a problem relating to blood sugar control and need to address their habits about 'sugar fixing'. For more information read *Chapter 5: Headache and migraine.*

Despite the perceived wisdom, child behaviour problems are hardly ever related to sugar consumption or the supposed 'sugar rush.' They are most often a reaction to cow's milk products or sweet artificial flavours, both which are often mixed with sugar. For more information read *Chapter 9: Child behaviour problems.*

Caffeine

How many of you think it would be better for your health to drink decaffeinated drinks? This is the word on the street, and every coffee shop provides them for their customers these days. Is that because caffeine is bad for you, or because if Café Nero sells decaff, Costa needs to do so as well, so as not to fall behind? Hmmm?

When I find coffee is a problem drink for any of my clients, their first comment will nearly always be, "Ah yes, the caffeine" with a sage nod of their heads. No! not caffeine, coffee! The coffee bean, not the caffeine.

The presumption is the caffeine in coffee, cola, tea, or chocolate is the problem, because caffeine is seen as bad for you. This has become a common perception because now every shop and café sells or markets decaffeinated drinks. Can it be that decaffeinated coffee is worse for you than normal coffee?

Certainly my figures suggest this, with 95% of regular decaff users in my 2015 Survey suffering symptoms from decaffeinated products...a huge percentage.

Decaffeinated drinks have been seen as a healthier alternative for decades now, but the chemicals and processes used to remove caffeine may be worse than drinking the tea or coffee which still contains caffeine.

Let us take a look at the history of decaffeination up to the present day. The use of the toxic chemicals benzene, chloroform and trichloroethylene was stopped back in the very early days of decaffeination. The next method used a chemical called dichloromethane. It was considered less toxic but its use was stopped in the 1970s when it was found to be carcinogenic. However, there are several common methods of decaffeination, which are still being used today.

The Chemical Solvent Method
Almost all decaffeinated coffee found in regular supermarkets and corner shops is processed this way. The common solvents used on the coffee beans include ethyl acetate, which is found in nail varnish and nail varnish remover and methylene chloride, found in paint stripper. The green coffee beans are moistened, soaked in the solvent, rinsed with water and then steamed.

The chemicals are supposed to be steamed out, but this was said of benzene back in the 1960s. Perhaps you can decide if tiny amounts of these chemicals are good for you in your regular coffee? Make a considered judgement as to why those of my clients who regularly drink decaffeinated products react adversely to the decaff when I test them, but not to the regular coffee or tea?

The Carbon Dioxide Method

In this method, the carbon dioxide actually looks like a liquid and is used at hundreds of times the normal atmospheric pressure. When the coffee beans are exposed to the carbon dioxide, the caffeine dissolves from the beans into the liquid. This appears to be a better method than the chemical solvent system, but unfortunately the product labelling does not state definitively which method has been used.

The Swiss Water Method

This method of decaffeination is different because it does not add chemicals to extract the caffeine. Beans are soaked in very hot water to dissolve the caffeine. The water is siphoned off and passed through a charcoal filter, which only holds the larger caffeine molecules, while enabling the smaller oil and flavour molecules to pass through. There are two end products:

- beans with no flavour or caffeine; and
- caffeine free highly flavoured coffee water [green coffee extract].

The flavourless caffeine free beans are discarded, but the flavour rich water is reused to remove the caffeine from a fresh batch of coffee beans.

Since this water is already saturated with strong coffee flavours, the flavours in this batch of coffee beans cannot dissolve into the water. Therefore, only the caffeine moves from the coffee beans to the water. The resulting coffee is decaffeinated without loss of flavour.

The Swiss Water Method is a safer and chemical free, decaffeination process. It is well labelled to distinguish it from the other methods.

If you do not sleep well, have high blood pressure, suffer palpitations, or feel wired or shaky when you drink several coffees, you need to reduce your intake of coffee rather than remove the caffeine. Otherwise, the Swiss Water Method is a good alternative and retains the flavour of the coffee bean better than other methods. Go for the Swiss Water Method, or reduce the coffee you drink to two or three mugs a day. If you are intolerant of the coffee bean, or tea leaf, you will need to cut out the drink completely. Intolerance is likely to build up to one of these drinks if you regularly consume three or more daily.

'Clean' eaters

There are many people I test who, as part of their way of life, read every article in every health magazine and know plenty about foods, vitamins and minerals. Their regular daily food and drink intake is very different from the majority of the population. Consequently, they are likely to become intolerant of completely different foods and drinks, because their frequent foods are different from the majority.

Case Study

Maya was a lovely 28 year old young woman who, having been part of the university and early twenties clubbing and drinking culture, made a sudden sea-change and decided she wanted to treat her body better. She read many health magazines and followed a huge number of suggestions around healthy eating. She went wheat and gluten free, with no tea or coffee, and she rarely drunk alcohol.

However, when she came to see me, her main symptom was throat clearing, which was something that had been occurring for many years in a minor way, but had increased to such a degree that it was becoming unacceptable. The throat clearing was driving her partner mad, it irritated him beyond belief, and he was nagging Maya to sort it out.

On testing, I discovered Maya was intolerant of:

- cow's milk products;
- green tea;
- coconut; and
- cassava.

As I regularly do, I started my session with Maya by explaining that the most likely foods to show up would be frequent, daily foods or drinks; foods she was likely to be using at least twice a day. When she was cow's milk intolerant I was not surprised. But Maya was! 'I 'don't really eat dairy' she stated. 'I think it is meant for baby cows not humans.' She ate pizza about once a fortnight and that was all. Historically though, Maya had eaten a lot of cheese and yogurt and I suspect dairy products had become a problem for her at that time.

Maya had read in many online articles, forums and in a multitude of health and fitness magazines that green tea is fabulous for you. She was especially attracted to it because of its low caffeine content, its high level of anti-oxidants, its cancer fighting properties and that it was mentioned so many times as being good for skin. She was drinking at least six cups daily, green tea extract was in her daily multivitamin and in the protein shake she used post gym workout three days a week.

In her quest for healthy living, Maya had sourced plenty of information about coconut oil, how good it is for your skin whether ingested or massaged. She told me of the many benefits she liked of using coconut, including that it:
- kills viruses bacteria, fungi, yeasts and parasites;
- improves digestion and absorption of nutrients;
- improves blood sugar regulation;
- helps protect against osteoporosis;
- improves digestion and bowel function;
- helps protect from cancer and is heart-healthy;
- helps prevent tooth decay;
- helps protect from free radicals as a protective anti-oxidant; and
- does not form harmful by products when heated.

Maya's favoured alternative for cow's milk was coconut milk. She regularly bought a coconut based vegetable curry for her lunch. She was using coconut oil instead of olive oil for cooking. Her diet was almost completely free of wheat and gluten. Nearly all of the alternative breads, cakes and flours she used contained cassava.

What showed up in her testing was all her problem foods were frequent foods/drinks for Maya. Not for most other people, but definitely for Maya. That is why she was reacting to green tea, coconut and cassava, regular foods and drinks, frequently used. Hmmm?

Why those foods?	Cause
Green tea	Frequency of use
Coconut	Frequency of use
Cassava	Frequency of use
Why then?	**Trigger**
We never worked out a trigger	

Maya's constant need to clear her throat ceased after about ten days on my suggested diet.

To recap
- The most common food intolerance additive does not even have an E number, it is sweet artificial flavours.
- Cow's milk intolerance is a much more common intolerance than all the additives added together.
- Decaffeinated products are not necessarily healthier for you than the regular tea or coffee.
- However healthy a food or drink is, an intolerance can build up when it is used regularly more than twice daily.

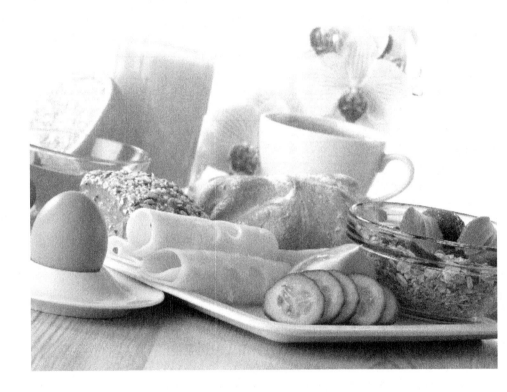

Part 4: Solutions

Chapter 15: Recommended diet for your age and gender

You may not be aware of the detail involved in giving up certain foods. Read *Chapter 16: Appendix* for details because avoiding staple foods is complicated. To be able to eat problem foods again, you need to avoid them completely for at least three months.

Adults and girls aged 16 +

Avoid the following foods for the first week.

Cow's milk products. Do not use other animal milks cheeses or yogurts as substitutes initially.

Yeast, all cheeses and all yogurts.

Cocoa if you eat chocolate daily.

Orange and grapefruit.

Tea or coffee if you use either drink more than twice a day, or if you have reduced your consumption from more than twice daily.

Decaffeinated drinks.

Any fruit if you eat or drink it twice a day or more.

Sweet artificial flavours if you consume sweets, fizzy drinks or fruit squashes daily.

Monosodium glutamate, E621 and other E numbers between E622 and E635.

Any drink or fruit you regularly consume more than twice daily.

Read the section on Withdrawal Symptoms later in this chapter.

When you feel better, which should be at the end of the first week, you could try any of the foods above, as it may be that several of them are alright for you. If you are managing the exclusion diet without too much trouble keep going on all the restrictions for the recommended three months.

Points to note
Less than 2% of the people I test are intolerant of both these major food groups:
- cow's milk products; and
- yeast, all cheeses, and yogurts.

It is very difficult to avoid both these food groups. As they are so rarely both a problem, I suggest you try each group in turn, to see which is your main problem. Eat bread to test yeast, if you feel fine, you only have to avoid cow's milk products for the next three months.

If your symptoms return, you need to avoid yeast, all cheeses and all yogurts for three months. Try some cow's milk, preferably just milk on cereal, or a glass of milk.

If the symptoms do not return then you can use milk, butter and margarine. Continue to avoid yeast, all cheeses and yogurts and the other drinks fruits and additives mentioned above for the next three months.

Males 16 - 18 years and all children under 16

Avoid the following foods for the first week.

Cow's milk products, plus milk, cheeses and yogurts from other animals, including sheep, goat and buffalo.

Orange in any form.

Cocoa.

Apple if eaten or drunk twice a day or more.

Other fruits, fruit juices or squashes if you consume that flavour twice a day or more.

Sweet artificial flavours if you eat sweets or drink fizzy drinks more than three times a week.

Monosodium glutamate and any E number between E621 and E635, if you eat instant noodles, pot noodles, crisps, gravies or stock cubes containing those additives a few times a week.

Aspartame if you drink sugar free or diet drinks daily.

Wheat if you are on the autistic spectrum.

Read the section on Withdrawal Symptoms later in this chapter.

Formula fed babies

For totally formula fed babies, problems will undoubtedly come down to the formula being used. Just about all baby formula milks are based on cow's milk. A cow's milk intolerance is extremely likely for any formula fed baby who is suffering adverse symptoms. If this is the case, you need to use a different formula. There are various options.

A formula based on soya, e.g. Wysoy. Soya formulas are not advisable for baby boys because of the high levels of oestrogen. If your baby is totally formula fed and having several feeds a day, there is always a possibility that he/she will develop an intolerance to soya from frequency of use.

A goat milk formula, e.g. Nanny Goat Formula. However, 50% of adults, children and babies with a cow's milk intolerance, also have a problem with goat, sheep and buffalo milks and that might not work for your baby.

Also, you need to consider frequency of use, because it is possible to develop another intolerance to any of these alternative milks.

You may be able to persuade your family doctor to prescribe **Nutramigen**, **Neocate** or **Alimentum formula milks**. These suit allergic babies very well.

Although I do not advise the use of a soya or goat's milk formula for more than a week, because of the possibility of developing an intolerance to that formula too, I recommend you try a soya formula for four or five days, just to see if your baby's symptoms can improve. Then go to your family doctor for advice and request a hypoallergenic formula milk such as Nutramigen, Neocate or Alimentum.

- If your baby is partially weaned, cut out all cow's milk products from your baby's diet. This is the most likely cause of any problems. Encourage your baby to drink water if you possibly can, as it will stop further problems arising with a fruit or fruit drink.
- Assess how often your baby eats something containing apple. Avoid apple if your baby uses it more than twice daily.

- To lower dependence on formula milks, encourage calories in the form of solids. Vegetables are rarely foods to which people become intolerant. Pureed vegetables, rice, oats and gradual introductions to meat and fish will help the potentially intolerant baby.

Breast fed babies

If your baby is totally breast fed, the breastfeeding mother needs to avoid the following foods for the first week.

Cow's milk products - do not use other animal milks, cheeses or yogurts as substitutes initially.

Cocoa if you eat and/or drink chocolate daily, or if you used to while you were pregnant.

Orange and grapefruit.

Tea or coffee if you use either drink more than twice a day, or if you have reduced consumption from more than two drinks daily.

Decaffeinated drinks.

Any fruit you eat or drink twice a day or more.

Sweet artificial flavours if you eat sweets, fizzy drinks and/or fruit squashes daily.

Monosodium glutamate E621 and similar additives including E622-E635.

Look in the Appendix for information about the above foods. Avoidance of these foods can be difficult and you will need good information.

- If your baby is partially weaned cut out all cow's milk products from your baby's diet. This is the most likely cause of any problems. Encourage your baby to drink water if you possibly can, as it will stop further problems arising with a fruit or fruit drink.

Point to note

The breastfeeding mother may feel unwell at the beginning of this exclusion diet because of withdrawal symptoms.

Withdrawal symptoms

Children rarely suffer withdrawal symptoms.

They are common in teenagers and adults.

When you stop eating a food or drinking a drink that you have been consuming all your life, or for several years, it is common to feel worse before you feel better.

Therefore, if you give up cow's milk products, an ingredient in bread, chocolate, tea or coffee, or anything you have been using regularly several times a day, it is expected that you will:

- suffer headaches;
- be irritable;
- feel tired; and
- suffer aching muscles.

It is normal to feel this way at the beginning of your elimination diet. Your symptoms may even initially worsen. Do not expect to feel better until about the fifth day of a diet change. The larger the total amount you have to give up, the worse you are likely to feel. If you are giving up a lot of tea, coffee, or cola drinks, it may make sense to cut down on frequency and amount used during a four or five day period. This will mean your withdrawal symptoms will not be so bad. Otherwise, the worst case scenario is that you suffer a blinding migraine or feel as though you have the flu and have to take to your bed.

If your symptoms are very severe, try eating or drinking one portion of your 'main' problem food, usually the one that you are missing the most. If you do not feel better within an hour, this suggests what you are suffering is not caused by withdrawing from that food.

Case Study

Jan had been suffering Irritable Bowel symptoms for many years and had just been 'putting up with it.' It was only when she started suffering from unexplained anxiety and palpitations that she sought my advice about food intolerance. Her heart had been investigated, and nothing abnormal found. She had also seen a counsellor privately, but was still spending most of her day in an extremely anxious state.

Withdrawing from the foods affecting her, sent her into a spiral of severe panic attacks within six hours. Her husband telephoned me, because he was really worried about her and was considering taking Jan to their local A and E. I recommended before he drove her there, to give her a cup of tea with milk, because these were the foods to which she was intolerant. If she felt better quickly, it would prove that these frightening symptoms were due to withdrawal from milk and most probably tea. She did feel better within ten minutes.

Bearing in mind that Jan was drinking six cups of tea daily for many years, I recommended she cut down on her tea consumption gradually during four days, rather than going 'cold turkey'. She did this and suffered only mild headaches. Four days afterwards, her anxiety was gone and her Irritable Bowel symptoms had settled.

Feeling no better?

If you or your child does not feel better on the diet I have recommended for you, you may be reacting to a food which less commonly leads to an intolerance. Consider some or all of the following foods and additives.

Soya

If you have been avoiding dairy products, are vegetarian or vegan, or regularly eat Japanese or Chinese food, soya may be something you use very frequently. Soya flour is also found in many breads these days. Soya might be the thing you regularly eat three or four times a day.

Sunflower
If you like seeded bread, cook with sunflower oil, eat sunflower seeds, muesli or granola, use a sunflower margarine or eat crisps frequently, sunflower is a frequent food for you.

Caramel E150-E155
Caramel is a dark brown/black artificial food colour. Read labels carefully on brown products and avoid this additive if you drink or used to drink a lot of cola drinks.

E471 Mono and Diglycerides of fatty acids.
E472 Esters of Mono and Diglycerides of fatty acids.
E282 Calcium Proprionate.

These are emulsifiers/preservatives commonly in bread and other baked goods, including: crumpets; muffins; cake; croissants; wraps; and soda bread.

If you are suspicious it is bread that causes you to suffer symptoms, avoid these preservatives as well. It might be these, rather than yeast or wheat that triggers your symptoms.

Coconut
If you use coconut frequently, because you believe in its health benefits, use coconut oil in cooking, regularly consume coconut milk or coconut water, regularly eat muesli or cereal bars, coconut might have become one of your most frequent foods.

Green tea, peppermint tea, chamomile tea
If you ignored my recommendations earlier concerning avoidance of any drink you consume three times daily or more, for example because you believe in the health benefits of green tea, please take notice of me now. Stop drinking any beverage if you use it three or more times daily.

Be aware that green tea extract is in many health and vitamin supplements and also in many protein shakes.

Reintroduction of foods after three months exclusion

After exclusion of food for three months, it is time to reintroduce each individual food individually, e.g. milk separately from cheese and yogurt, cocoa, orange etcetera at four day intervals. If you have five foods to introduce, this will take about three weeks.

Please do not take this stage too quickly, because certain foods will be alright and others might not.

For each food, eat or drink a reasonable portion on two consecutive days. During the next three days watch for any adverse symptoms. This is because certain symptoms, especially joint, back and neck pain and depression, can take a few days to kick in, anything up to three days.

If no adverse symptoms occur, it will be alright for you to eat or drink these items in moderation.

Here are my guidelines regarding **moderation** for the different food groups, guidelines which I have developed during the last 15 years of advising clients.

Cow's milk products
When you can tolerate milk, cheese and yogurt on two consecutive days without adverse symptoms, do not go back to your original pattern. Your normal intake was too much for you before and it will be too much for you again. You will risk redeveloping the intolerance.

Count all cow's milk based products as one family of foods, even a small amount in butter, margarine, tea or coffee, and have no more than two portions daily. Only eat cheese twice a week. It will help if you keep using alternative milks in the medium term, or learn to take your hot drinks black, to keep your use of cow's milk products low.

Yeast, all cheeses and all yogurts

Yeast counts as one portion whether it is a large amount, e.g. in bread, or a small amount, e.g. in stock cubes or flavoured crisps. Use yeast once daily as a maximum and only on four days in an average week. Cheese only twice a week. Yogurt one portion on only four days a week.

Cocoa

Twice a week maximum, evenly spaced through the week...never two days running.

Orange

Twice a week maximum, evenly spaced through the week...never two days running.

Tea, coffee or any drink you were taking frequently

Once or twice a day maximum. If you do not like the taste after three months exclusion, nature is telling you something. You are not ready to use these drinks yet. Try again in a month.

Any other food or additive

Use it 50% less frequently than you did when you were regularly eating/ drinking the item.

I developed these client guidelines because I found that unless restriction is maintained, clients come back to be retested because they have redeveloped their original food intolerance. Keeping to these guidelines has meant very few people return for testing and they are able to manage their own condition, while still being able to eat relatively normally.

To recap

- Three months exclusion is essential.
- Adults usually suffer withdrawal symptoms.
- Careful reintroduction of foods is advised.
- Any food or drink consumed twice or more daily could be something that you are intolerant to.
- Do not go back to your original patterns of eating after three months exclusion. You risk redeveloping the intolerance.

Appendix

APPLE

Avoid apple in any form.

Apples	Apple juice
Apple squash	Mixed fruit juices will often contain apple
Mixed fruit squashes will often contain apple	Smoothies will often contain apple
Apple is often mixed with blackcurrant	Check pickles and chutneys
Apple pie	Apple crumble
Apple is sometimes used to sweeten soya milk	Apple is in many baby foods
Apple pieces and apple peel are in most fruit teas	Check fruit, bars and cereal bars for apple
Apple is used to sweeten some rice cakes	Some wholesome childrens sweets are 100% apple juice
Apple is in some gluten free breads	Apple cider and apple cider vinegar

ASPARTAME [E951]

Aspartame is the most commonly used artificial sweetener.

It is commonly in these products. Sometimes a different sweetener such as sucralose is used.

Diet drinks	Sugar free, low sugar or no added sugar squashes
Sugar free mints and chewing gums	Low fat yogurts

Flavoured waters	Artificial sweetener tablets or powders
Berocca, and chewable vitamin tablets	Low fat or diet savoury products e.g. Weightwatchers baked beans, Dolmio Lite
Alcopops e.g. Smirnoff Ice, Bacardi Breezer	Protein shakes

CARAMEL [E150 - E155]

This is labelled colour [caramel], colour [ammonia caramel] or colour [caramel sulphite]. Caramel is a dark brown/black artificial food colour. Check ingredients on all products that are pale brown to black in colour.

It will be in all of these products.

Gravy	Cola drinks and cola bottle sweets

And might be in these products depending on the brand.

Soy sauce	Oyster sauce
Brown sauce	Barbecue sauce
Stock cubes and stock gels	Flavoured crisps
Fudge	Toffees
Cheap chocolate	Caramel sweets
Mocha frappes	Some gluten free breads

CHROMIUM SUPPLEMENTATION

Chromium is needed in your diet to aid blood sugar control.

Symptoms of chromium deficiency
When your blood sugar is low because you have not eaten for too long, you will suffer the following symptoms.

Headache	Irritability
Nausea	Shaky
Sugar craving	

How to keep your blood sugar more stable.

Eat frequently	Do not use sugar to raise your blood sugar
Eat more complex carbohydrates (whole grains)	Eat more protein
Take a chromium supplement	

Research the GL [Glycaemic Load] diet.
Research the GI [Glycaemic Index] diet.
Every food has a Glycaemic Index, which is an indication of how well it can keep your blood sugar stable.

Supplement dosage
Chromium 200-400mg daily.

COCOA

Avoid chocolate in any form.

Chocolate bars	Chocolate cake
White chocolate	Chocolate/choc chip biscuits
Nutella	Dark chocolate
Chocolate mousse	Chocolate desserts
Coco pops	Chocolate milkshakes
Hot chocolate	Mocha drinks
Chocolate in cappuccinos	Sometimes in liquorice
Cacao	

Cocoa is also in some savoury foods.

Chilli con carne	Beef casserole
Packet mixes for chilli con carne	Some beef gravies
Some flavoured crisps	Sauces for chilli con carne

CHEMICAL FRAGRANCE

Can contribute to, and in some cases be a major part of the picture, with the following symptoms.

- Headache, migraine, nausea, asthma, rhinitis, catarrh, sneezing, wheeze, cough, throat clearing, sinus problems, ear problems, tinnitus, if inhaled.

If you suffer from these symptoms, please do not use the following.

Air fresheners	Plug-in air fresheners
Pot pourri	Fabric conditioners
Fabric softeners	Fragranced candles
Cheap perfumes	Cheap after-shaves

Incense sticks	Fragranced diffusers
Fragranced bleach	Fragranced cleaning sprays and polishes

The products below do not usually cause problems with these symptoms.

- Flash with bleach
- Cif no fragrance
- Dettol or Dettox no fragrance
- Lord Sheraton, Pledge Original or Mr Sheen Original furniture polishes

CHEMICAL FRAGRANCE AND COLOUR

Can contribute to, and in some cases be a major part of the picture, with the following symptoms.

- Skin rashes, eczema, psoriasis, itching, if present in washing, bathing or moisturising products.
- Dandruff, flaky scalp, psoriatic scalp, cradle cap, itchy scalp, itchy ears, itchy face, facial rash, eczema or rash on hands, if in shampoos or conditioners.

If you have a skin condition, be aware that nearly all the regular clothes washing products will aggravate your skin, as do normal soaps, shower gels, shampoos. Please do not even use non-bio products, and definitely never use fabric conditioners.

If a product is fragranced, NEVER USE IT.

If a product has a colour to it, NEVER USE IT.

The product needs to be white or clear in colour, to not adversely affect your skin.

The products below do not usually cause skin symptoms.

- **Surcare:** washing products for clothes washing. But do not use Surcare fabric conditioner. It makes some people itch.
- **Aveeno:** products.
- **Simple:** soap, shower gel, shampoo, conditioner, moisturizer and sun cream.
- **Simple and Aveeno products:** suit most people with skin issues, but are unsuitable for some. If they do not work for you, source a natural product that is colour and fragrance free.

Follow all these instructions. To 'cherry pick' what is easy for you will not get the best results.

COMMON FOOD INTOLERANCE SYMPTOMS IN ADULTS

Headache	Irritability
Eczema	Migraine
Mood swings	Rash
PMS	Itch
Abdominal pain	Concentration problems
Psoriasis	Wind
Anxiety	Acne
Diarrhoea	Panic attacks
Acne Rosacea	Loose stools
Depression	Constipations
Mouth ulcers	Indigestion
Behaviour problems	Itchy mouth
Reflux	Nausea
Aching joints	Sore eyes
Vomiting	Aching muscles
Fibromyalgia	Sleep problems
Catarrh	Back pain
Nightmares	Rhinitis
Neck pain	Night sweats

Sneezing	Gout
Cough	Rheumatoid arthritis
Throat clearing	Asthma
Fluid retention	Fatigue
Frequent colds	Lethargy
Cystitis	Thrush
Athlete's foot	

COMMON FOOD INTOLERANCE SYMPTOMS IN CHILDREN

Headache	Irritability
Mouth ulcers	Migraine
Mood swings	Itchy mouth
Concentration problems	Infantile colic
Behaviour problems	Sore eyes
Tummy aches	Attention Deficit Disorder
Wind	Hyperactivity
Sleep problems	Diarrhoea
Oppositional Defiant Disorder	Nightmares
Loose stools	Dyslexia
Constipation	Night sweats
Indigestion	Reflux
Itchy bottom	Bed wetting
Nausea	Thrush
Vomiting	Cystitis
Fatigue	Athlete's foot
Lethargy	Catarrh
Eczema	Croup
Rash	Dark shadows under eyes
Rhinitis	Sneezing
Itch	Cough
Psoriasis	Throat clearing
Frequent colds	Asthma
Growing pains	Aching tired legs

COW'S MILK PRODUCTS

Read every list of ingredients, and ask questions of staff in restaurants. You will be amazed at where milk can be hidden. Never trust eating anything until you have read all of the ingredients.

In the UK and EU food labelling system, milk is highlighted, capitalized or boldened, e.g. MILK, **milk**. Any product that states 'may contain milk' will be alright for you unless you have an allergy to milk.

Avoid the following.

Cow's milk	Cow's cheese
Cow's yogurt	Lactose
Buttermilk	Albumin
Casein	Whey
Lactalbumin	Caseinate
Butter	Margarines
Cream	Crème fraiche
Yogurt probiotic drinks	Doughnuts
Scones	Yorkshire pudding
Pancakes	Crossaints
Pizza	Quiche
Caesar Salad	Baileys liqueur
Most pesto sauces	Coffeemate and powdered milks
Chocolate	Toffee
Fudge	Butterscotch
Mousses	Milky sauces e.g. lasagna, carbonara
Custard	Ice cream
Whey protein shakes	Creamy puddings e.g. cheesecake, trifle

Milk may be in these foods. Some of these items you will be surprised at, make sure you read labels on everything that you eat or drink.

Bread, especially sweeter bread like buns, brioche	Mayonnaise and salad cream
Curry	Battered or breaded products
Biscuits	Some cooked meats, e.g. ham, chicken pieces, chorizo, pepperoni
Gravy powders or granules	Some artificial sweetener tablets
Some vitamin and mineral tablets	Many medicines, including the contraceptive pill
Some flavoured crisps	Homeopathic remedies in pill form

ALTERNATIVES FOR ANIMAL MILK PRODUCTS

Milks

Soya milk	Rice milk
Oat milk	Almond milk
Hazelnut milk	Coconut milk
Hemp milk	

Cheeses

Coconut cheeses	Soya cheeses
Rice cheeses	

Yogurts

Coconut yogurts [Coyo, Coconut Collaborative]	Soya yogurt [Alpro]

Margarines

Dairy free margarine [Pure, Vitalite, Stork hard margarine]

Ice-creams

Soya [Swedish Glace, Tofutti]	Cashew [Booja-Booja]
Coconut [Booja-Booja, Coconut Collaborative]	Almond [Almond Dream]

Chocolate

Dark, bitter chocolate [Green and Black's, Lindt 85%]	Sweeter milk free chocolate [Moo-Free]

Sheep's, goat's and buffalo products

You may not have a problem with other animal milks, cheeses and yogurts. When you are feeling better, try sheep's, goat's and buffalo products and see how you feel. 50% of people with a cow's milk intolerance can tolerate other animal milks, but many will suffer similar symptoms to those they had with cow's milk.

Do not use any alternative food, e.g. soya, coconut, sheep's or goat's milks more than twice a day, to prevent new intolerances developing.

MONOSODIUM GLUTAMATE E621

Monosodium glutamate is a savoury artificial flavour enhancer.

It is mainly in 'junk' food. Poor quality ingredients are used, and the nicer flavours are enhanced by the addition of monosodium glutamate.

It may be found in the following foods.

Cheap Chinese food	Many Chinese sauces
Flavoured crisps	Packet soups
Instant noodles	Flavoured couscous
Flavoured rice	Cup-a-soups
Dry roasted peanuts	Bombay mix packet snacks
Gravy powders and granules	Cheap meat pies
Some pasties	Savoury flavoured rice cakes
Stock cubes	

In the last five years, a new raft of monosodium glutamate look-a-likes have been chemically produced. Products containing these chemicals can all legitimately say that they are MSG free, and this has proved a very good selling point. Their E numbers are very close to MSG, and they seem, for many people to give the same symptoms as MSG.

Their E numbers and names are as follows.

E622 Monopotassium L glutamate	E623 Calcium diglutamate
E624 Monoammonium glutamate	E625 Magnesium diglutamate
E626 Guanylic acid	E627 Disodium guanylate
E628 Dipotassium guanylate	E629 Calcium guanylate
E630 Inosinic acid	E631 Disodium inosinate
E632 Dipotassium inosinate	E633 Calcium inosinate
E634 Calcium 5ribonucleotides	E635 Disodium 5ribonucleotides

ORANGE

Avoid the following.

Oranges, satsumas, mandarins, clementines, pomelos	Orange juice and squash
Tropical juice and squash	Orange marmalade
Orange peel [in fruit cake, fruit teas, mince pies]	Cointreau and Grand Marnier liqueurs
Smoothies	Orange lollies
Orange sorbets	Orange sweets

When someone is intolerant to orange, grapefruit may well give similar symptoms, but lemon, pineapple and lime rarely do.

You may use citric acid, as these days it is a chemical unrelated to the citrus in oranges.

PANIC ATTACKS

Symptoms
You will feel that you cannot breathe. You will look and feel frightened. Your heart will be racing. You may complain immediately or later on that you have tingling in your fingers or arms, or that your hands feel strange.

Reasons for symptoms
If someone is anxious or very nervous about something, the hormone called adrenaline is released. This is the one that copes with 'fight, flight or fear'.

Thousands of years ago this was very useful for running away from a tiger, but we do not need that these days!

Blood is needed to get to the muscles quickly to enable the person to run really fast, therefore heart rate increases. Oxygen is needed because if you run fast you get puffed. Therefore, there has to be an increase in breathing rate.

In the absence of being able to run fast, the oxygen is not required. If you over-breathe for a while, you get too much oxygen in your blood. This has the effect of making hands and arms tingle and feel weird. This is frightening, therefore panic increases. It is a vicious circle.

Action you need to take
- Try to remain calm. You need to practise these strategies when you are not in the throes of a panic attack. Can you get a buddy to help you? Someone who might be around when you panic? Friend, partner, work colleague?
- Use a paper bag or a large envelope.
- Breathe in and then breathe out slowly into the paper bag. Continue breathing in and out into the paper bag...slow breaths...breathe in to the count of six and then out to the count of six.
- Do six breaths like this, then one of normal air. Continue until symptoms go away. This means that you will eventually be breathing in a higher concentration of carbon dioxide, which will reduce the symptoms.
- Concentrate your focus on your breathing, and on something in your environment.
- Count dots, lines, panes of glass in a window, leaves on a tree...

It really does help to think to yourself about adrenaline, tigers, oxygen, carbon dioxide, if you can because then you can understand what is going on.

You can understand your symptoms, and that reduces panic

It can take twice as long to lose the symptoms of panic as it took to build up in the first place.

If you fight it for ten minutes it will take 20 minutes to go away.

Cognitive Behavioural Therapy [CBT] can be very helpful.

SOYA

British and EU regulations stipulate that soya in products must be highlighted, boldened or capitalised in lists of ingredients. [e.g. SOYA, soya]

Avoid the following.

Soya bean	Edamame bean
Textured vegetable protein	Tempeh
Tofu	Soya milk
Soy sauce	Soya yogurt
Soya margarine	Soya desserts
Soya flour	Soya lecithin

Soya flour is in many breads and other baked goods e.g. cake, buns, doughnuts. Soya flour makes a very soft light bread or cake.

Breads that tend not to contain soya flour are as follows.
- Ciabatta
- Part-baked loaves
- Pitta bread
- Crumpets
- Artisan breads

SUNFLOWER

Sunflower, in various forms, is in many foods.

Sunflower seeds can be in the following.

Cereal bars	Muesli
Granola	Seeded bread
Seeded crispbread	

And sunflower oil can be in the following.

Margarines	Cereal bars
Granola	Crisps
Oven chips	Potato wedges

Also avoid sunflower lecithin, an emulsifier.

SWEET ARTIFICIAL FLAVOURS

Read ingredients on any sweet products, including the following.

Sweets	Desserts
Chocolate	Fizzy drinks
Jellies	Yogurts
Fruit squashes	Probiotic drinks
Protein shakes	Jam
Childrens medicines	Cereal bars
Breakfast cereals	Flavoured waters
Ice cream	Cake
Syrups in coffee shops	Amaretto
Muffins	Doughnuts
Buns	

Avoid any products which contain 'flavour' or 'flavouring'.

'**Natural**' flavour or flavouring will not be a problem.

'**Flavouring**' in savoury products will not be a problem.

Alternatives
- **Fizzy drinks** - 7up, Appletiser, Peartiser, Grapetiser.
- **Sweets** - Fruitella, Natural Confectionary Company, some Rowntrees sweets.
- **Yogurts** - Yeo Valley, Rachel's Organic, Onken, Coyo, Coconut Collaborative.

COFFEE
Avoid all coffee including decaffeinated, plus coffee cake, coffee sweets, Tia Maria, tiramisu.

TEA
Avoid all tea including decaffeinated, earl grey, lady grey, darjeeling, green tea, black tea, white tea, rooibosch, chai, lapsang souchon.

Green tea extract is often included in vitamin supplements and protein shakes.

Alternative hot drinks include the following.

Camomile tea	Barleycup
Peppermint tea	Caro
Fruit teas	Dandelion coffee
Nettle tea	Bambu
Hot squashes	Teecino
Cinnamon and cardamom tea	Lemon and ginger
Fennel tea	Lemon and honey

Be careful not to have more than two cups of any flavour daily, or you might become intolerant to another drink.

TYPICAL SYMPTOM CHANGES IN FOOD INTOLERANCE

Baby with colic, vomiting or posseting, sleep difficulty or eczema.

Toddler with eczema, asthma, constipation, diarrhoea, catarrh or glue ear.

Primary school age child with headaches, tummy aches or asthma, catarrh or glue ear.

Teenager with headache, migraine, abdominal migraine or IBS.

Adult with IBS, headaches, catarrh, joint pain.

A food intolerant person can suffer from many symptom changes through their lifetime.

VITAMIN A SUPPLEMENTATION

Symptoms of Vitamin A deficiency include the following.

Acne	Allergies
Sore gritty eyes	Poor night vision

Supplement dosage
Beta-carotene 15mg daily

Do not exceed stated dose of Beta-carotene. Do not supplement with vitamin A.

VITAMIN B6 SUPPLEMENTATION

Symptoms of vitamin B6 deficiency include the following.

Headache	Migraine
Pre-menstrual syndrome	Depression
Anxiety	Irritability
Acne	Behaviour problems
Concentration difficulties	Learning disabilities
Fluid retention	Sometimes weight gain

Supplement dosage
Vitamin B complex with 80-100 mg daily in the mornings. Make sure supplement is yeast and milk free.

Side effects
- Numbness in fingers or toes [only noted on 200mg dosage]. If you get these symptoms, reduce the dose or discontinue.
- Luminous yellow urine.

YEAST - ALL CHEESES AND ALL YOGURTS

When yeast is part of your food intolerance picture, you will find that there is a problem also with all cheese, and all yogurt. Avoiding only yeast will not help you.

You need not avoid natural yeasts in wine, or brewer's yeast in beer. Most peoples' reactions are to baker's yeast...the sort that is in bread and the other items mentioned below.

Avoid the following.

Bread	Rolls
Croissants	Bagels
Crumpets	Buns

Pizza	Naan bread
Pitta bread	Sourdough bread
Flatbread	Pretzels
Breaded items	Taramasalata
Flavoured crisps	Stock cubes
Gravy powders and granules	Many vegetarian products
Marmite	Bovril
Vegemite	Soups
Some vitamin and mineral supplements	

Bread alternatives include the following.

Soda bread	Tortilla wraps
Ryevita	Oatcakes
Corn crackers	Rice cakes
Some wheat crackers	Scones
Cake	

CHEESE

Avoid all cheeses, cow's, sheep's, goat's, buffalo, cheddar, brie, ricotta, mascarpone, cottage cheese, edam, paneer, cream cheese, mozzarella, vegan, vegetarian, including the following.

Pizza	Quiche
Fromage frais	Cheesecake
Pesto	Lasagne
Carbonara	Tiramisu
Cheesey biscuits	Cheese and onion crisps
Paninis	Caesar salad
Carrot cake icing	Some fruit mousses

YOGURT

Avoid all yogurts, cow's, sheep's, goat's, soya, coconut, low fat, 0% fat.

Yogurt is found in the following.

Some curries	Some naan breads
Yogurt dips	Yogurt probiotic drinks
Goulash	Some fruit mousses
Yogurt coated nuts, raisins or cereal bars	

If you suffer from thrush, athlete's foot or other fungal infections frequently, read about candidiasis in *Chapter 11: Wheat intolerance. Myth, fact or yeast?*

ZINC SUPPLEMENTATION

If you have any of the following skin problems, or behaviour or concentration problems, you will benefit from supplementing zinc.

Eczema	Rash
Itch	Psoriasis
Dermatitis	Acne

Supplement according to the chart below.

0-6 months	3mg daily
7-12 months	4mg daily
1-3 years	5mg daily
4-8 years	7mg daily
9-13 years	10mg daily
14-18 years	15mg daily
Adults	30mg daily

Zinc dosage is normally in 15mg tablets. Make sure the supplement is milk and yeast free.

For dosages less than 15mg, you can buy zinc drops from www.biocare. co.uk.

Index

A

Acne 18, 23, 44-46, 64-69, 71-73, 146,157-158, 160

Addiction 62-63

Additives 20, 22, 24, 34, 87, 103, 106, 110-112, 117, 121, 127, 131-132, 135, 137-138, 140

Air fresheners 53, 57, 60, 62, 75-76, 144

Alcohol 20-21, 27-28, 43, 56, 102, 107-108, 118-120, 125

Antibiotics 13, 26, 69, 107-108,

Anxiety 15, 44, 46, 80-81, 83-84, 98, 137, 146, 158

Apple 27-28, 34-35, 37-38, 43, 47-48, 53, 65, 86, 132-133, 141

Artificial flavours 155

Aspartame 27-28, 34-35, 38, 43, 87, 91-92, 132, 141

Asthma 23, 35, 74-77, 79, 85, 144, 147, 157

Attention Deficit Disorder 87, 89, 147

Attention Deficit Hyperactivity

Disorder 87, 89

B

Beer 118-119, 158

Behaviour problems 85, 87-89, 91, 93, 122,146-147, 158

C

Beta-carotene 46, 68-69, 72-73, 157

Blackcurrant 34-35, 38, 54, 91-92, 116, 141

Bloating 23, 40-41, 48, 71, 101, 113, 119

Bread 18, 29-30, 44-47, 56, 61-62, 81, 101-103, 105-106, 127, 131, 136-138, 140-142, 149, 154, 158-160

Cassava 126-127

Catarrh 13, 18, 23, 74-79, 85, 144, 146-147, 157

Cheese 27-30, 36, 42-43, 45-46, 52, 59, 65, 69-70, 72-73, 81, 88, 91, 97-98, 101-102, 104-108, 115, 126, 130-132, 135, 139-140, 148-150, 158-159

Children 13, 21, 23, 27-28, 30-31, 34-35, 37-38, 43-44, 53, 64-66, 74-75, 78, 86-92, 110, 114, 121, 132-133, 136, 147

Chocolate 28-30, 45, 48, 53, 56, 58, 61-62, 69-70, 73, 83, 86, 101, 115-117, 122-123, 130, 135-136, 142, 144, 148, 150, 155

Chromium 52-53, 55-57, 59, 61-63, 90, 115-116, 143

Chronic Fatigue Syndrome 83

CPSIA information can be obtained
at www.ICGtesting.com
Printed in the USA
LVOW04s1730210916

505621LV00018B/1181/P